MANAGING
HEALTH SERVICE
INFORMATION SYSTEMS
An Introduction

MANAGING HEALTH SERVICE INFORMATION SYSTEMS
An Introduction

Edited by
Rod Sheaff and Victor Peel

Open University Press
Buckingham · Philadelphia

Open University Press
Celtic Court
22 Ballmoor
Buckingham
MK18 1XW

and
1900 Frost Road, Suite 101
Bristol, PA 19007, USA

First Published 1995

A catalogue record of this book is available from the British Library

ISBN   0 335 15702 5 (pbk)   0 335 15703 3 (hbk)

Library of Congress Cataloging-in-Publication Data
Managing health service information systems : an introduction / edited by Rod
  Sheaff and Victor Peel.
     p.   cm.
  Includes bibliographical references and index.
  ISBN   0–335–15702–5 (pbk.)   ISBN   0–335–15703–3 (hb.)
    1. Medical informatics—Great Britain.   2. National Health Service (Great
  Britain) I. Sheaff, Rod. II Peel, Victor. 1947–   .
    [DNLM 1. Information Systems—organization & administration. 2. Medical
  Informatics Applications. W 26.5 M266 1994]
  R859.2.G7M36 1994
  362.1'068'4—dc20
  DNLM/DLC
  For Library of Congress   94–27219
                                                                                  CIP

Typeset by Type Study, Scarborough
Printed in Great Britain by Biddles Ltd, Guildford and King's Lynn

CONTENTS

LIST OF FIGURES
AND TABLES

THE EDITORS AND CONTRIBUTORS

Simon Aldridge is contracts and business manager at South Manchester Community NHS Trust. His PhD at Manchester Business School studied the implementation of health service information systems.

Norman Ambage is head of information at the Macclesfield District General Hospital, East Cheshire NHS Trust. He has been involved in health service information for over six years, much of that time as a provider unit information manager. He has been responsible for raising awareness of information issues within general and clinical management circles and for raising the profile of information team work in the hospital environment. Currently he is involved in implementing his trust's information strategy. This involves helping to procure and implement a HISS, developing a strategy for community information systems and working with managers in developing the use of information to support general and clinical management.

Roger Dewhurst is head of regional information services for Mersey Regional Health Authority, and a director of the Health Care Consultancy and the software division of CSL Limited. He has extensive experience of working with both NHS providers and purchasers in implementing the NHS reforms. His earlier career was within both local authorities and the private sector, specialising in the use and development of graphical information systems.

Chris Mackintosh works with a consortium of fundholding general practices in Bristol, using information systems to inform their healthcare purchasing. A geography graduate from Bristol University, he was for seven years a civil service soil hydrologist in working in the UK and abroad, before becoming information manager in general practices in Chester and then Castlefields Health Centre, Runcorn.

Lorraine Nicholson is a fellow in health service management and a member of Oldham Family Health Services Authority. Her work includes a number of projects for the National Health Service Management Executive. Since 1992 she has undertaken significant projects for the Audit Commission, including an evaluation of the English medical record system and has been involved in the NHSME Data Quality Review in six NHS Regions. She has advised many healthcare organisations outside the UK on health and medical records policy.

Victor Peel is head of the centre for health informatics at the Health Services Management Unit, University of Manchester. Formerly general manager of Bolton Health Authority, he now advises many NHS bodies, the NHS Management Executive, many overseas health organisations, a number of information system producers, and the World Health Organisation on policy and management in healthcare information and technology.

Caroline Rea is a fellow in health service management at the Health Services Management Unit, University of Manchester. A prize-winning MBA student at Henley, her career in the NHS culminated in the post of resource management project coordinator at Guys Hospital, London, having previously been a business manager for renal services there. Her activities centre upon working with clinical directorates, providing development support for clinical directors and business managers and undertaking consultancy and teaching with a number of organisations which have adopted the clinical directorate model of management.

Gina Shakespeare works for the NHS Womens Unit of the NHS Management Executive. A member of the Institute of Health Services Managers, she has published widely in the *Health Services Journal, Medical Annual* and other healthcare publications.

Rod Sheaff joined the Health Services Management Unit at the University of Manchester in 1984 after posts in operational management and with the Department of Health. He has published widely on health policy, ethics and marketing. He is the author of *Marketing for Health Services*, the first British book on the subject and has worked extensively in both the British and a number of overseas health care systems.

Heather Walker joined the Health Services Management Unit as a Fellow in Health Records in 1989. Graduating in social studies from Newcastle University, she joined the NHS as a Regional Administrative Trainee in Mersey Region. Her managerial experience within the health service was spent as Health Records and Patients Services Managers in several acute units, including two large teaching hospitals. Besides directing management development programmes for medical records managers, healthcare professionals and women managers she has evaluated medical records tenders for Greater Glasgow Health Board, reviewed the use of Read Clinical Classifications for Yorkshire Regional Health Authority and completed data quality reviews in six regions. She is now participating in the Audit Commission review of medical records in England.

PREFACE

Developments in both informatics and health service management pose the question of how health services can exploit new information technologies in the 1990s. This book tries to address the question, outlining in Chapter 1 a sequence of stages for introducing or modernising a health service information system, starting from the objectives of the health service organisation itself. Following this sequence, the book aims to give health service managers and other health workers (including clinicians) having little previous experience of health service information systems enough knowledge to work with information and technology staff to introduce, manage and use a modern healthcare information system. This does not involve the type of technical knowledge required to attempt, say, dataflow diagramming or software debugging for oneself. Our aim is to give enough familiarity with principles and technical developments for the clinician or a managerial generalist to recognise where he or she requires expert help, what help is required, and how to use and be critical of (rather than simply depend upon) the inevitably partial viewpoints of enthusiasts or salesmen. This includes an understanding of the connections between information systems and the underlying objectives of health services themselves.

We therefore emphasise the organisational aspects of health information systems more, and the technical less, than many informatics texts do. The book dwells particularly upon what Chapter 1 calls the preselection and selection phases of information system implementation, starting (in Chapters 2–5) at organisation-wide level. Then the focus shifts to individual service levels (Chapters 6–9). Chapters 7, 10 and 11 examine the actual implementation and installation of a healthcare information system. We finish (in Chapter 12) by assessing the longer term implications of internal markets for health service informatics and suggesting some proposals for health service information policy, research and development. In all this we have drawn largely on British National Health Service experience but many of the principles and lessons have a wider application.

We gratefully acknowledge the help given by Al Dowling, Valerie Ferguson, Andrew Haw, Jeff James, David Kwo, Karin Lowson, Bruce Neumann and Christina Thomson; and thank Jacinta Evans for her forebearance in waiting for a script that took some time to come to fruition. Besides contributing much of the text, Heather Walker took on the role of managing editor. Without her, the text might never have materialised.

LIST OF ABBREVIATIONS
AND ACRONYMS

AAH Meditel	[proprietary GP information system brand name]
A&E	Accident and emergency (department)
ACORN	A Classification of Residential Neighbourhoods
AMRO	Association of Health Care Information and Medical Records Officers
APG	ambulatory patient group
ASCII	American Standard Code for Information Interchange
ASSIST	Association of Information Management and Technology Staff in the NHS
ATT-ISTEL	[proprietary hospital information system brand name]
BASIC	Basic Programming Language
BCS	British Computer Society
BMA	British Medical Association
BS	British Standard
CASE	Computer aided software engineering
CAT	Computer assisted tomography
CDAM	*Catalogue des Actes Medicaux* (catalogue of medical treatments – France) [coding system]
CEPIS	Council of European Professional Informatics Societies
CEPOD	Confidential Enquiry into Perioperative Deaths
CIMA	Chartered Institute of Management Accounting
CISP	Community information system for·purchasers
CHC	Community Health Council

CMDS	contract minimum data sets
CMMS	case mix management system
COBOL	[a programming language]
CPHA	Commission on Professional and Hospital Activities (USA)
CPT3	Current Physicians' Terminology (version 3)
CRIR	Committee for the Review of Information Requirements
CSL	Computer Services Limited
CSSD	Central Sterile Supplies Department
dBASE	[proprietary database brand name]
DFD	dataflow diagram
DHA	District Health Authority
DHSS	Department of Health and Social Security
DIN	doctors' independent network
DISP	developing information systems for purchasers
DMIS	[proprietary decision support system brand name]
DNA	'did not attend'
DRG	diagnostic related group
DSON	Detailed statement of need
ECR	extra-contractual referral
ECT	electro-convulsive therapy
EDI	electronic data interchange
EDIFACT	Electronic Data Interchange for Administration, Commerce and Transport
EIS	executive information system
EL	executive letter
E-mail	electronic mail
EMEDI	European medical data interchange (standard)
EPR	electronic patient record
ETHICS	Effective Technical and Human Implementation of Computer based work Systems [methodology]
EU	European Union (formerly European Community)
EU-GATT	European Union – General Agreement on Tariffs and Trade Regulations
FDL	finance directorate letter
FHSA	Family Health Services Authority
FPC	Family Practitioner Committee
GP	General practitioner
GPFH	General practitioner fundholder
GPAS	[proprietary Scottish GP administration system – brand name]
GOSIP	Government Open Systems Interconnection Profile

HA   Health Authority
HAA   hospital activity analysis
HC   health circular
HCIMO   *Adaptation Hospitaliere des Maladies et des Operations*
                (Hospital Version for Illnesses and Operations –
                Belgium) [coding system]
HELP   [proprietary hospital information system brand name]
HIPE   hospital inpatient enquiry
HISS   hospital information support system
HIW   health information workstation
HL7   Health Level 7 [protocol]
HRG   Health resource group
HSMU   Health Services Management Unit, Manchester
                University

ICCS   International Classification of Clinical Services
ICD(+ number)   International Statistical Classification of Diseases and
                Causes of Death (+ revision number)
ICD-9-CM   International Classification of Diseases, Ninth Revision,
                Clinical Modification
ICU   intensive care unit
ICWS   integrated clinical workstation
IFHRO   International Federation of Health Records
                Organisations
IHSM   Institute of Health Services Management
IMG   [see NHSME-IMG]
IM&T   Information management and technology
INAMI   *Institut National d'Assurance contre la Maladie et
                l'Invalidite* (National Institute for Sickness and Invalidity
                Insurance – Belgium) [coding system]
IOCR   intelligent optical character recognition
IP   in-patient
IS   information system(s)
ISAC   information system work and analysis of changes
                [methodology]
ISO   International Standards Organisation
IT   information technology

JANET   Joint Academic Network
JICNARS   Joint Industry Committee for National Readership
                Surveys
JSD   Jackson Systems Development [methodology]

LAN   local area networks
LOTUS   [a spreadsheet brand name]

MAAG	Medical Audit Advisory Group
MCI	Management Charter Initative
MDU	Medical Defence Union
MEDICINE	Medical Data Interchange (project)
MEMPHIS	Measuring and Economic Modelling of the Performance of Healthcare through Information Systems
MNTK	*Mezhotraslyevoi Nauchno-Tekhnicheskii Kompleks* (inter-sector scientific-technical complex – Russia)
MPI	master patient index
MS-DOS	Microsoft Disc Operating System [proprietary brand name]
NAI	non-accidental injury
NHSAR	National Health Service Administrative Register
NHSIS	National Health Service Information Systems
NHSME	National Health Service Management Executive
NHSME-IMG	National Health Service Management Executive Information Management Group
NHSTA	National Health Service Training Authority
NHSTD	National Health Service Training Directorate
NLSO	Nordic List of Surgical Operations [coding system]
NMIS	nurse management information systems
NVQ	National Vocational Qualification
OCS	order communications system
OPD	outpatients department
OPCS	Office of Population Census and Surveys
OPCS4	Office of Population Censuses and Surveys Classification of Surgical Operations, Version 4.
OR	operational research
OSI	open systems interconnection
OS2	Operating System 2
PACS	picture archiving and communications systems
PACT	Prescribing Analysis and Costs Tables
PAS	Patient Administration System
PC	personal computer
PEST	political, economic, social and technological (marketing analysis)
PET	positron emission tomography
PHIS	Public Health Information Specification
PI	performance indicator
PMC	Patient Management Category
POISE	Procurement of Information Systems Effectively
PRINCE	Projects in a Controlled Environment [methodology]
ProPAC	Prospective Payments Commission (USA)

QALY	Quality-adjusted life year
RAWP	Resource Allocation Working Party [formulae]
RCGP	Royal College of General Practitioners
RCS	Royal College of Surgeons
RHA	Regional Health Authority
RIP	renal intensive care programme (software)
RMI	Resource Management Initiative
RMO	resident medical officer
ROI	return on investment
ROM	read-only memory
SAPPHIRE	System Accreditation Project for Primary Healthcare Information Requirements and Evaluations
SASP	Summary Analysis of Strategic Plans
SHSL	[Filing code for official notifications to FHSAs]
SID	Strategic Intent and Direction (Welsh NHS)
SIP	Sickness Impact Profile
SNOMED	Systematized Nomenclature of Medicine
SSADM	Structured Systems Analysis and Design Methodology
STRADIS	Structured analysis, design and implementation of information systems development methodology (brand name)
TDS	[proprietary hospital information system brand name]
THESAM	*Thesaurus des Archives Medicales* (Medical archive thesaurus – France) [coding system]
THIS	total hospital information system
TQM	total quality management
UCDS	uniform clinical data sets
Unix	[an operating system brand name]
VAMP	[GP information system brand name]
VAN	value added network
VESKA	*Vereinigung Schweizerischer Krankenhauser* (Union of Swiss Hospitals) coding system
WAN	wide area network
WHO	World Health Organisation
WL	waiting list
WORM	'write once, read many'
X400	[a communications standard]

Chapter 1

INFORMATICS AND HEALTHCARE

Rod Sheaff

Health service Informatics in the 1990s

Information is a resource as necessary for the effective provision of health care as trained staff, adequate buildings and equipment. British health service administrators began to perceive this in 1974, but the perception has been sharpened considerably by the onset of health system reform in Britain, in other European countries and the USA. These reforms are *inter alia* responses to pressure to contain costs of health care. Since cutting health budgets is unpopular and demand for health services is increasing, governments have tried to increase health system activity through administrative reform and resource reallocation rather than by budget increase. A precursor and corollary of larger reform, this 'strategy of managerialism' attempts to professionalise health services management and to model it increasingly overtly on private sector commercial management. Commercialisation of healthcare is a policy objective in much of Europe, comprehending both the public expenditure containment and the managerialist strategies. In Britain, France, the Netherlands, Sweden and parts of eastern Europe (e.g. Romania, Poland, Russia) more radical health system reforms are leading towards various forms of 'internal market' (Mordelet 1992; Rado 1992; Ministry of Health, Education and Welfare 1992). There are even discussions in Germany about patient co-payments (Anon 1992). Meanwhile there has been a revitalisation of public health through the *Health for All 2000* and its national counterparts (*Health of the Nation*, in Britain) (WHO 1984; Department of Health 1991). This requires epidemiological databases for targeting, managing and monitoring innovations in public health (e.g. breast screening). Partly for these reasons and partly for cost-containment reasons, economic and technical evaluation of clinical practice is becoming a more common (though not yet everyday) activity for health services managers. One result of all this is the necessity for more sophisticated management information systems in the National Health Service (NHS).

Another is the politicisation of healthcare, which in the United Kingdom has led governments to require increasing amounts of data to legitimise and (less often) to ground health policy. An example would be the Citizens' Charter target of having no patients waiting more than two years for their first outpatient appointment by April 1992. To demonstrate success in achieving this target, in time for the 1992 general election, required the aggregation of the data from routine administrative systems, and identifying from the list of patients waiting over two years as many as possible who had died, not joined the list through the correct procedure, moved house or 'gone private' so that they could be excluded from the figures (Mullen 1992).

These events pose new requirements for health service information systems, increasing the sheer volume and complexity of managerial data to collect and analyse. In character, scale, complexity and purposes, health service information systems will continue to change radically and rapidly during the 1990s. These changes originate more in the demands of health policy – hence health service management, and hence the role of information systems within the wider healthcare organisation – than they do in information technology. Nevertheless, developments in information technology (IT) and informatics, in computer and communications systems, software and hardware make it possible to restructure, enlarge and automate health service information systems ever faster and more cheaply. These technical developments originated largely in the military, space and academic sectors and have spilled over into other sectors (including health) since the 1960s.

Furthest-reaching has been the development and popularisation of microcomputers, sustaining an industry which rightly sees the health sector as a large market. Miniaturisation of computers down to desktop, now palmtop, size through microchips has increased their portability and range of applications (e.g. in intelligent medical instrumentation and autoanalysers). Developmental work is in hand to replace mainframe data storage systems with linked phalanxes of cheaper, smaller desktop hard discs. This suggests an extreme geographical mobility of administrative functions will become possible as administrative work becomes more computer-based (Ernst & Young 1989). There is a trend towards ever higher performance specifications in storing, combining and analysing data, in carrying out many operations (analyses, collations, printing, etc.) simultaneously, faster and on a larger scale. Falling equipment prices are another consequence of miniaturisation, and mass production. Market-leader microcomputers (say, the Apple

2 in 1980, IBM-compatible personal computer (PC) 'clones' now) have become cheaper in cash (let alone real) terms since 1980, and the lower price buys a higher-specification machine.

A certain standardisation of equipment, programs and methods of networking machines has followed the popularisation of microcomputers but commercial interests have obstructed the trend. The ideal competitive strategy for, say, a microcomputer firm would be to invent and patent its own equipment, operating systems, etc., which outclass existing systems but which other firms cannot imitate or produce compatible alternatives for; and then get these systems accepted as market or industry or official standard. Even IBM, however, failed at this strategy (*L'Express* 1991). Its recent collaboration with Apple suggests that the non-standardisation between these two market leaders in the microcomputer market will gradually be palliated.

New managerial applications of computerised information systems continue in the non-health sectors. Computer aided design and computer integrated manufacture are increasingly being used to accelerate the product lifecycle, reducing the time lag between someone having a new product or service idea and the actual introduction of the new commodity in the market (Ernst & Young 1989). Use of management information systems to support strategic business planning is becoming more common. In some sectors the market itself has been automated, for instance with airline ticketing and some financial markets (Ernst & Young 1989: 10). Some of these innovations (e.g. automated booking systems) have obvious health service uses.

A most important characteristic of the new information technologies is their flexibility and adaptability. Standard hardware (e.g. an IBM compatible PC) has many applications. Many applications software packages are available as turnkey systems for common, standard uses (e.g. word processing) and many of these software packages can be adapted locally by users themselves. Even the process of software adaptation and design has been automated ('CASE' – Computer Aided Software Engineering) (Ernst & Young 1989: 7, 24). Ancillary technologies such as bar-coding and digital recording of images have developed alongside.

These developments present health services with both an opportunity and a problem. The opportunity can be outlined by explaining why managing information systems is important; its applications and benefits, in descending order of importance to health service users.

For the health service user the purpose of health services is to keep him or her well and, when that fails, to provide what cure, or failing that what care, is attainable. Health service efficacy, and consequently information about it, is required at three levels. At population level, it contributes to maintaining health through intersectoral activity, promoting healthier personal behaviour, and providing preventive health services. At purchaser level the central task is to ensure access and availability of health services for those who need them. Here an important role of information is to ground and legitimate claims and decisions on resources. At provider level the critical questions are those of service efficacy, efficiency and quality for the individual patient or client. This includes evaluating the quality of care and innovative forms of care, both for clinical outcome and (where different) for the psychological and social quality of life for clients, patients and informal carers. All three levels concern health service purchasers. Service providers are primarily concerned with the third, health promoters with the first.

Information on all three levels is also required for advancing health policy debates, and raising their level so that health policy discussions are based more upon data and less upon politicians' and journalists' fantasies. Well-designed information systems can be used to show when health service successes or failures reflect causes outside the health system, or the design strengths or weakness of particular services, or just individuals' peculiarities. Managing health services, especially through an internal market, poses obvious information requirements: to support health authorities' (HAs') buying decisions and contract monitoring (see Chapter 3), and to support provider business planning and marketing (see Chapters 5 and 12) will require much more rapid responses that hitherto in increasingly unstable settings. Two of Roy Griffiths' criticisms of NHS information systems therefore had point: the dearths of outcome, quality, consumer data (and *a fortiori* NHS managers' ability to respond to it) and of cost information (insofar as the health system is monetarised) (Griffiths 1984).

The NHS has a glut of underanalysed data. The question is, how to use information systems to harness it. Three types of application are emerging. Clinical and technical applications are most obvious. They include expert systems such as the renal intensive care programme (RIP) – software for managing intensive-care renal patients. For routine clinical management they already include automated warning and monitoring systems, e.g. health risk appraisal systems (WHO 1988: 50), bedside monitoring systems, non-accidental injury (NAI) registers and so on. Teleradiology (remote hospital analysis of electronically communicated X-ray images) and other picture archiving and communications systems (PACS) are becoming available (Kropf 1990; Allison and Martin 1993). Statistical process control is already used from some industrial processes in UK hospitals (e.g. in central sterile supplies departments – CSSDs) and it is only a matter of time before it is applied to the commoner, simpler clinical procedures. At least one German hospital and one English hospital have experimented with doctors carrying palmtop computers for calculations and technical reference.

Automating existing patient administration (both management and clinical aspects) is the second type. In 1992, the first UK experiments began with a view to implementing electronic patient records (EPRs). Automation allows both greater access and confidentiality, greater flexibility (e.g. by putting health records into patient-held smart cards) and wider health records linkage. There is also increasing scope to automate and simplify clerical work such as routine wordprocessing, billing, and pharmacy records, releasing staff for more skilled activities. Some industrial information system developments, such as computer assisted design, have direct healthcare applications, for instance in hospital building design or the design of prostheses. Automated booking and planning systems can allow better use of vehicles, staff and other resources.

Decision support systems are the third type of application, and for managers the most important because of the contribution they make to developing the health system: for supporting decisions on innovating new forms of health service, discovering more rational (not only cheaper) forms of service (e.g. substituting hospice for acute hospital care) and giving a better factual basis from which to appraise existing practice. Service innovations are especially likely to result from combining information technologies. For example combining database with communications technology has yielded computer assisted learning and distance learning (e.g. via satellite links, through media such as EuroTransMed) and databases on current research findings and good clinical practice (e.g. Medex, Medline, both very underused in the United Kingdom). An obvious application is to network health record systems district health authority (DHA)-wide, even nationally (WHO 1988: 48), supporting integration of primary, secondary and tertiary care. This would be the best (though not the only possible) basis for the faster, more complex analyses of trends and correlations of health data (length of stay trends, referral and discharge analysis, case mix, clinical audit summaries, etc.) that automated information systems offer. Realistic modelling of the internal market, service and epidemiological changes, by spreadsheet or simulation methods, then becomes possible. NHS organisations started attempting this in the 1980s with models such as Sargeant Troy (on manpower planning), Burdwall (on estates management) and Rubber Windmill (a business game simulating the regional level of the NHS internal market). In the 1990s more sophisticated models for simulating hospital activity have become widely used.

The problems can be explained by briefly outlining the history of NHS information systems. Farther-sighted health service managers began exploring the above possibilities some years ago. Four stages of development are discernable in UK NHS information systems. Until 1976 there was only the administrative collection of data, through local, manual systems. Financial accounting systems were centralised but there was little localised budget holding at, say, department (or in some cases even hospital) level. There was virtually no automation. Limited attempts were made from the late 1960s to apply operational research (OR) methods in designing 'productivity' pay deals. In retrospect, the most significant event may have been the Tunbridge report on medical records (see Chapter 8). The NHS planning system and Resource Allocation Working Party (RAWP) necessitated centralised collection of the data on service provision used both to calculate norms and assess services against them. Standardised planning forms such as Summary Analysis of Strategic Plans (SASP) were invented, worked manually, with some support from mainframe computing at regional level. The latter was also used to automate some clerical functions such as payroll preparation. From this period dates the emergence of 'health service statistics'.

As cash-limited budgeting spread down the management hierarchies in the early 1980s, NHS financial systems became increasingly automated at district level. Efforts to compare information on the management of NHS districts at regional level and centrally led to the Körner Report on health services information (DHSS 1982) and the first Performance Indicator (PI) packages. Meanwhile the WHO produced its first report on health service information systems. Free-standing microcomputer-based systems began to appear, introduced mainly by clinicians for clinical and research purposes. By now the importance of information as a resource in its own right had been recognised by many health authorities and such jobs as 'District Information Officer' were appearing. These developments tended to occur more and faster in acute health services than in primary or community care or health promotion.

With the internal market reforms announced in 1989 information has taken a new significance, as one of the most important means by which purchasers are to manage the market and monitor provider compliance with service contracts. Yet NHS information systems are most developed for clinical management and medical records purposes, or for automating clerical routines. Not only is informatics least developed in the area of managerial decision support systems but the type of decisions which require information support (and hence the information required to support them) have suddenly changed. Meanwhile healthcare information technology continues to develop autonomously and at an accelerating pace, increasing the capacity to meet many of these new requirements.

Some spectacular débâcles in implementing NHS information systems (e.g. the Wessex and West Midlands Regional Health Authority (RHA) procurement scandals, the collapse of the London ambulance control computer system (Mullin 1992)) show that realising this potential is not easy. Many health service managers (including health professionals in their managerial capacities) find themselves having to operate or introduce information systems without knowing what sort of information system to order; nor how to install and operate it; nor what sort of information to demand of the system; nor how to use it for decision support. This book tries to address these questions. To begin it is necessary to explain what informatics is, and to outline some principles of information management.

What informatics is

Healthcare informatics develops at the junction of healthcare management, economics, accounting, clinical practice, and information technology. Unfortunately this means it is infested with jargon from each. Yet the technical terms are briefer and more exact than everyday language. Understanding an inescapable minimum of terms is necessary preparation for the chapters that follow. This section explains some main concepts and principles of healthcare informatics (fuller explanations are in general informatics texts such as Ball *et al.* 1991, Burch and Grudnitski 1986, Quinn 1992 or Szymanski, Szymanski et al. 1988). Terms are *italicised* where they are explained below.

First must be the term *informatics* itself. According to the World Health Organisation (WHO):

> Informatics may be defined as the combination of technology and methodology which makes possible the computer-assisted collection, storage, processing, retrieval, distribution and management of information. (WHO 1988: 3)

Some writers use the word 'informatics' for the developing body of theory, information science, which explores such questions as the relation between information technology and information systems and between information systems and organisation structure; others for the actual equipment and systems themselves. Either way, some terms used here require explanation in turn.

The term *information technology* tends to be associated with computer- and telecommunication-based, automated information handling. This is too narrow. Any technique for recording data, analysing it into information and presenting it is an information technology. Technologies have two aspects: physical resources (raw materials and tools); and knowledge about these resources and how to manipulate them to achieve specific results (Woodward 1965; Engels 1975).

As physical tools nearly all information technologies have hitherto used simple, manual resources; pen, print, paper and filing systems which have changed little since the early industrial period. The familiar medical (or health) record systems are 'the most important tools for information storage and retrieval, and analysis of health care' (WHO 1988: 47). Manual technologies, however, typically produce only inaccurate and incomplete information, and can only handle limited data volumes and analyses (WHO 1988: 18) because data collation, transmission, storage and analysis is laborious, slow and expensive. In automated information technologies the physical tools are the hardware and networks. *Hardware* is the physical equipment required by the information systems. This is pen and paper in the simplest manual systems; in automated systems it is keyboards, screens, modems, processors, printers and storage media (hard and floppy discs, tapes, optical compact disc or other forms of 'read-only memory' (ROM).

Telematics, or *communications*, is the use of electronic means to transmit data and programs between computers. Such systems of links, whether using special wiring or telephone circuitry, are called networks. *Networks* are the means by which dispersed parts of the information system communicate with each other; in automated systems the wiring, terminals, modems (modulator-demodulators, for converting computer signals into forms that can be transmitted by phone lines intended for voice), telephone lines and exchanges, fileservers and spoolers. Examples include JANET (Joint Academic Network) for file transfer between universities. *Local area networks* (LANs) connect computers and other equipment, such as printers, in different parts of the same workplace. Often using their own special wiring, LANs are usually limited to distances of a few hundred metres by the electrical characteristics of the computers and the network. *Wide area networks* (WANs) overcome this distance limitation. A special type of WAN is the *Value added network* (VAN), where the network is used to distribute saleable data or information. Videotex methods (e.g. Viewtex, Prestel) do this through the telephone system, Ceefax and similar methods use television transmission.

Electronic mail (E-mail) is an increasingly important use of networks. E-mail uses a computer terminal (a microcomputer or a special screen and keyboard) to produce a letter, memo or other document to transmit to one or many terminals simultaneously where it can be read as it arrives or stored until the addressee uses the machine. E-mail allows free formating of text – use of any page layout, spacing or sequence of information – just as an ordinary letter does. *Electronic data interchange* (EDI) differs in using standardised forms which lend themselves to routine transactions such as automated requisitioning or billing.

Besides the physical resources, technologies include technical knowledge. In the case of information systems. this knowledge consists of understanding the data and information that the hardware stores, communicates and analyses, and of the software and supporting theory which record how the hardware does this.

One difference between information technology and other technologies is that the raw material of information technology is not something physical, but data. Information is produced by collecting, processing and interpreting data. Information is produced from data, but raw data do not usually constitute information. *Data* are, literally, 'givens'; the raw, brute-empirical pieces of knowledge given in uninterpreted, unanalysed form (or as near as one can get) in the 'real world' (Avison and Fitzgerald 1988: 6). Epistemologists dispute exactly how 'raw' or 'uninterpreted' data can ever be but in informatics data are treated as the most objective, irreducible, veridical form of knowledge available to an information system. Data can be quantitative (e.g. 73 129 outpatients in X hospital in 1992) or qualitative (e.g. patient's sex: male). In practice, data are usually grouped, stored and communicated in data files. However, a single set of data alone does not necessarily give a rounded, exhaustive picture of the state of affairs a manager or researcher wants to investigate. Without proper interpretation, even raw data can be partial or misleading (80 per cent of patients seen within 10 minutes of booked appointment times might seem a high level until one discovers that an older, less well-staffed neighbouring hospital achieves 85 per cent). Neither do data necessarily indicate any practical judgement. The datum that patient X waited 55 minutes to see his doctor simply reports an event. Whether the outpatients department (OPD) manager should worry about this waiting time or congratulate herself depends on its relation to other facts and to managerial policy or objectives (e.g. how this wait compares with waits in other clinics or with *Patients' Charter* standards).

Analyses convert data into information. They are the processes by which information systems summarise data, draw conclusions, and present the summaries and conclusions in intelligible and practically useful forms to the system user. So what counts as data, and what as information, is context-dependent; one person's information is another's data (Avison and Fitzgerald 1988: 6). Average waiting times in a given clinic would be information for the clinic manager but data for the hospital manager comparing waiting times in different hospitals' clinics. A common type of summary is to collate data elements. A *data element* is a piece of data which, with other such pieces, builds up into a meaningful overall picture of a particular problem or situation – for instance an individual patient's clinical condition (Irvine 1990: 15); which then serves the doctor as data for his or her clinical decision making. Another common method of analysis reveals or exploits *data structure*: the relationships holding among a collection of data (e.g. correlations between variables, definitional connections between them). Data structures can therefore change over time as correlations between different pieces of data change (e.g. as the relationship between patient diagnosis and normal referral route changes). Yet another common analysis is filtering: 'Data are filtered through summarizing and classifying operations that screen out unnecessary detail for a given level of decision making' (Burch and Grudnitski 1986: 54).

Mediating between hardware and networks on one hand, and the data and analyses on the other, is the system software, without which the hardware is unusable. *Software* is the coded instructions making the hardware operate as, say, a wordprocessor, a data storage system, the control unit of another machine, or in some other capacity. Software is structured in different levels. Directly corresponding to the on-off switching of electric circuits within a microchip is machine code, written as a series of '1's and '0's. Sometimes this binary code is summarised into hexadec code (using base-16 numerals) but the next important level is that of the *operating system* which consists of instructions telling the hardware which data or programs to load, which disc, printer or other equipment to use, and which basic operations (e.g. reading, writing) to perform. At present, a few rival operating systems (e.g. OS2, Unix, MS-DOS) are contesting to become standard. Languages (e.g. BASIC, COBOL) consist of standardised commands making the hardware do more complex operations (e.g. mathematical calculations, comparisons).

Programs are sets of instructions using a language, operating system and machine code to make the hardware function as word-processor, database, statistical calculator or other machine. *Applications* and macro programmes take a generic, standard programme (e.g. LOTUS spreadsheets) and config- ure it for a particular use (e.g. as an accounting spreadsheet). *Turnkey* programs are standard, ready-to-run programs for which the user has to do little more than load the program into the computer and follow instructions (often they come with an operating system built in).

Specialised organisations often require specially written software and configurations of equipment for their information systems. By 'method- ology', informaticians mean 'methods for devising an information system for a particular application' – a special case of project management. These are methods for analysing how part of an organisation, production process or service works in order to yield a model of the data flows involved, from which software writers can make a system design. Tailor-made software can then be written, or a suitable ready-made system bought. Different *methodologies* include Effective Technical and Human Implementation of Computer-based Work Systems (ETHICS) (see Chapter 7), Structured Systems Analysis and Design Methodology (SSADM – already used in the NHS; see Ashworth and Woodland 1990), Projects in a Controlled Environment (PRINCE – also in NHS use; see Burdess 1993) and Jackson Systems Development (JSD). There are textbooks which explain these methodologies (e.g. Downs et al. 1991; Mumford 1994; Mumford and Wier 1979; Jackson 1983). Different methodologies often share some techniques of which one, dataflow diagram- ming, is illustrated in Chapter 6.

The point of modernising an organisation's information systems is to make its working practices faster, more flexible, or more effective in meeting its objectives. Information systems do this in two ways. *Office automation* consists of automating routine work (in health services, this includes clinical and general administration). *Decision support systems* provide information to support decision making. The decisions supported may be routine (e.g. clinical management decisions at individual patient level) or non-routine (e.g. policy, strategic and research decisions). The difference is illustrated when cost reduction is a motive for automating an information system. Whether office automation can be expected to save running costs depends on local circumstances. Staff savings may accrue from large-scale automation of administrative routines (e.g. billing, patient bookings), but against this costs rise for telephone line use, equipment maintenance, consumables (discs, specialised stationery), modified buildings, etc. All these costs constitute the opportunity cost of the information system as a whole. Opportunity cost is standardly defined as the benefit foregone by automating the information system instead of putting the resources to their most productive alternative use:

> Because resources are scarce we are forced to choose. A choice means that you have one thing or the other . . . If by cost we mean what must be given up in order to obtain something then the cost of having more bread is having less of something else . . . The economist's term for expressing costs in terms of foregone alternatives is OPPORTUNITY COST'.   (Lipsey 1970: 60–1)

Nevertheless, office automation often does raise productivity or reduce costs, although health service managers are sometimes over-optimistic about how much (Peel et al. 1993). In contrast, decision support systems usually generate productivity gains or savings, if any, only indirectly by creating the capacity to review previously under-managed services. If such gains occur, however, they are often large. For example, a new system in an English RHA revealed patterns of lengths of stay for cataract removals that enabled day surgery to replace a three- or four-day inpatient stay for most patients. The time and money savings for hospitals, and perhaps also for patients, did not result directly from the decision support system but would have been impossible without it.

Of greatest interest to health service managers are *management information systems*: decision support systems for managers, which have two main uses. A monitoring use consists of reporting, summarising and analysing current, 'live' data on what has actually happened in or to the organisation. The other is generating hypothetical data from the real data; *modelling* or making projections to answer 'what-if?' questions about what will happen if a given trend continues or if a certain decision is made. For instance a hospital manager might use such a system to predict the effects of a changing patient case mix on mean length of stay, throughput, variable costs, staffing levels and operating theatre capacity.

What type of information systems an organisation requires therefore depends heavily on what work it does and on what decision support its managers require. All this depends on the organisation's objectives. In the case of healthcare these objectives in turn depend largely on its place in the health system as a whole, indeed in the whole social system. This has practical implications which the next section explores.

The early life of a health service information system

Since the purpose of a health service information system is to serve its organisation's objectives, these are the necessary starting points for deciding how to build or modernise a health service information system. It is nearly

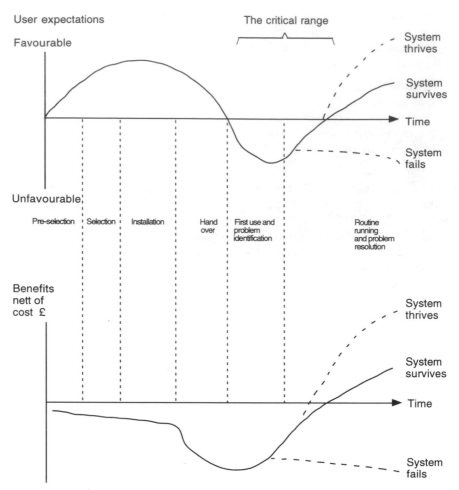

Figure 1.1   Changing expectations, costs and benefits of an information system
Source: Adapted from material by A. Dowling

always a mistake to start (as computer sales staff prefer) by considering what equipment to buy. A rational sequence for modernising an information system (Figure 1.1) has five stages, equipment being purchased only at the end of the second stage.

Following chapters concentrate on those phases of the cycle requiring a specifically managerial input: the preselection and selection phases, the implementation aspect of the third phase, and the problem-resolution aspect of the fifth stage if especially severe problems arise. Chapters 3 to 6 concern the all-important preselection phase, and Chapters 8, 9 and 11 the selection phase, leading to the choice of hardware and software. Chapters 7 to 11 also deal with installation, problem solving and routine running – the handover of a working system to line managers – above all on the organisational or 'implementation' aspects. Other aspects of healthcare information systems are primarily tasks for technical experts although managers need to know enough about them to monitor progress and anticipate any major difficulties. This section uses the sequence to explain further concepts arising from the WHO definition of 'informatics' (continuing to italicise technical terms which require explanation).

Preselection consists, first, in identifying what information the system should generate for decision support purposes. These requirements should be minimised, or at least ranked in priority order, partly to focus on producing the most practically necessary information, partly because data production has an opportunity cost. These requirements will normally include descriptive summaries of data (e.g. total patient throughput for a whole hospital each week), breakdowns of data (e.g. throughput by speciality, ward or doctor), and analytic statistics (e.g. projections of throughput over the next year, correlations between throughput and length of stay). All this gives a first approximation to decisions on how data are to be collected, updated and worked up into information. Because management information systems are used first to decide practical targets, formulate them and monitor achievement preselection also requires deciding who is to receive what information and for what purposes.

All this depends upon articulating the organisation's objectives explicitly. The latter may already be stipulated in policy documents (e.g. business plans) but more usually they will have to be articulated through discussions with senior managers and, in health services, clinicians. Once formulated, these objectives (e.g. 'to maximise health gain') have to be operationalised (i.e. translated into definite, specifiable) targets. For financial or activity objectives this is comparatively easy but to operationalise real health objectives, indicators of health status or of healthcare outcome have to be selected or devised. This is a specialist task in itself, and a number of texts now explain what validated indicators are already available and what issues have to be addressed in devising new indicators (Bowling 1991, Holland 1983, Sheaff 1991: 73–9).

A corollary of re-articulating the service's objectives is to formulate the purposes and uses of its information system by specifying what contribution to these objectives the information system is to make. This is the important and often neglected preliminary to *benefits realisation* (cf. NHSME-IMG 1992a). The manager should state precisely what contribution to the organisation's objections the information system is to make, so that it will later be possible either to demonstrate this has occurred or analyse why it did not (a UK example is Peel 1993). Benefits may be defined in terms of the organisation's objectives, activities, beneficiaries or cost. WHO policy itemises a 'family' of information systems, suggesting that information systems can contribute at the levels of policy making, detailed service programming and budgeting, monitoring and control of health policy information, and evaluation and reprogramming of healthcare (WHO 1988: 16–7). In a commercial health service the corresponding question might be: will a new information system be required to generate an identifiable return on investment (ROI)? If so will this ROI be the same as that required for other capital projects? (WHO 1988: 11).

Preselection is, thirdly, the time at which to decide how far the new information system must satisfy external bodies' demands. These include deciding how far the new system is to:

1 Be compatible with information systems outside the health sector (e.g. is it desirable to be able to exchange data with the national census or local government?), hence able to update itself in line with developments there (WHO 1988: 6, 8).
2 Be a means, in publicly owned health systems, of supporting the local IT industry.
3 Adopt ISO9000 (International Standards Organisation Standard 9000) or standards stating ethical and legal requirements on civil liberties and data security. In the UK, these requirements include the Data Protection Act, patient access to (most) health records, maintaining health records for legal purposes (recording consent, sectioning, post-mortems, etc.). This may include political acceptability. There was opposition to creating national patient databases in post-war West Germany.
4 Meet WHO, European Union (EU), central government, Department of Health and (in the British NHS) National Health Service Management Executive (NHSME) requirements for information; and, in the case of providers, purchasers' requirements for information for contract monitoring and payment purposes.
5 Interface with other information systems at health system level (regional, national, or international bodies, databases, etc.); at organisational level (e.g. interfacing a clinic's information systems with that for the whole hospital); and at service level (e.g. whether to network wards with laboratories and operating theatres).
6 Allow public access, for instance (in the NHS) to data on levels of performance and maximum waiting times (as suggested in the *Patients' Charter*) and, conversely, to know what types of confidentiality must be guaranteed.

A strategy for introducing and disseminating the new information system is also best decided at the preselection phase (see Chapter 2). One aspect is the choice of type of system: for instance what kind of *Total Hospital Information System* (THIS), called in the NHS a Hospital Information

Support System (HISS), to aim at. A THIS is normally an *order entry results communication system*, which automatically generates and sends orders for tests, blood, food etc. on-line between hospital departments. An *open architecture* THIS consists of localised, specialised information systems each dedicated to one task (e.g. databases and monitors for blood or tissue matching, or systems controlling complex equipment such as computer assisted tomography or CAT scanners), with distributed processing but networked hospital-wide. A *closed architecture* THIS consists of a single, centralised system (Gale 1993). Either strategy will have to specify which parts of the information system to build first and why, and whether to build onto existing information systems such as those already developed for resource management in parts of the British NHS. As with any capital project, the strategy has to anticipate when, and under what conditions, a decision on whether to extend the information system would be taken; in the worst case, at what point would the new information system be written off as a failure; and what are the limits on the time and money that can be spent on the system?

An *information management strategy* can also be decided at the pre-selection phase. It states who will undertake the detailed design, installation, management, repair and modernisation of the information system. For a hospital or community service the main options are to:

1 Make each department be responsible for its part of the information system (perhaps with unit-wide technical support).
2 Give one existing department (e.g. quality assurance or finance) responsibility for managing information for all other departments.
3 Create a new department for information (if this should be done, should it incorporate the medical records service?).

In a small health service organisation such as a general practice, the corresponding question is whether the practice manager or one of the partners should introduce an information system, or whether outside advice should be bought in.

A standards strategy is also best decided at this stage. It specifies what data definitions, communication standards or other technical specifications must be adopted throughout the information system to allow for future net-working, for unit-wide (or wider) aggregations, comparisons and analyses of data, and for data exchange. Here the word 'standards' is used in an informatics sense not the more familiar sense associated with quality assurance. Information *standards* stipulate what data will be collected and how, the technical specification and performance of software, what protocols will be followed (see below), the methods of working (on confidentiality, etc.), equipment performance, the content and quality of training, and the ethics and technical competences of information workers (WHO 1988: 14).

Where patient safety will depend on the timeliness, accuracy and availability of data it is particularly important to set standards for data *backup* (i.e. routinely making duplicate copies of data) and prepare contingency procedures for breakdowns in the information system.

Such standards allow compatible equipment and software to be bought from different suppliers, and are a precondition in turn for networking and telematics. Standard data definitions allow comparability and common understanding of data, terminology and the information produced from them. They save each information system from reinventing basic technical solutions to problems of (e.g.) software design. They simplify software maintenance and modification, and the purchasing and installation of information systems. They can be used to guarantee minimum levels of data security (WHO 1988: 10), and allow system providers and users to write consistent, intelligible and up-to-date documentation that is easier to modernise as the system develops (WHO 1988: 10, 65). Use of standards enables staff to transfer their training between different organisations. Even if the choice of standards be left to technical experts it is for the manager to ensure that standards are chosen and then adopted uniformly throughout the hospital or service.

A *systems analysis* culminates the preselection phase. It shows the overall structure of the proposed information system in terms of what types of data will be generated, when and how they will be collected, how they will be stored, how updated, how presented and to whom. The essence of systems analysis is clear grasp of the purposes of the information system, which is why the previous activities of the preselection phase are necessary. The usual starting point is a systems analysis of the existing, often manual, information system. Systems analysis is often done by flowcharting the existing systems, using a standard set of symbols or (in the NHS) by following the relevant parts of SSADM. The initial systems analysis is then modified in light of the requirements decided upon in the preselection phase (see above). Then the detailed technical design and procurement of the information system can begin.

The *selection* phase begins with production of a detailed *systems design* derived from the systems analysis. A system design is a technical design of an information system meeting the objectives identified in a systems analysis (Burch & Grudnitski 1986: 461). Main steps in systems design are to (Burch and Grudnitski 1986: 482):

1 Review the information system's objectives.
2 Evaluate any constraints on what systems are possible.
3 Design the output (i.e. what information will be produced, how presented).
4 Design a model showing what data analyses, breakdowns, summaries, etc. will produce the output.
5 Input design, stating how data will be put into the information system.

6 Design the controls: tests to ensure the information system meets user specifications, including specifications for security and data accuracy.
7 Plan system installation.
8 Cost the new system.

This text treats system design as a task primarily for the informatician or software expert. *Data flow diagrams* (DFD) are often produced at this stage. Chapter 6 includes one (Figure 6.1). Using standardised symbols a DFD maps the design of data collection, processing and output flows in the proposed information system.

By this stage some more technical decisions can be made. They include *data definitions* stipulating how data will be categorised. For instance: for costing or staffing reasons hospital managers often wish to know how many beds a particular service uses. The problem then is, what counts as a bed? Beds on a ward or intensive care unit (ICU) obviously count, but do trolleys in day surgery units, couches in delivery suites, beds on one ward being 'borrowed' by another, or beds used by NHS patients in a private hospital? Valid inter-speciality or inter-hospital comparisons in terms of beds require a common definition of the term 'bed': and this is its data definition. Data standards stipulate how timely, accurately and completely data are to be collected for analysis or inclusion in the reports produced by the information system.

Protocols, also chosen at the selection phase, define how data and instructions shall be coded and formulated by information systems to allow the data and instructions to pass between them. ASCII (American Standard Code for Information Interchange) is an example. It defines how numbers, letters, signs and some machine commands shall be translated to and from the binary code required for electronic storage and transmission. A protocol adopted for a publicly funded health service in Europe should fall within the Open Systems Interconnection (OSI), a generic 'reference model' which accommodates a range of protocols (including ASCII). OSI is endorsed by the International Standards Organisation (ISO). The EU, ISO and UK government recommend a functional profile called GOSIP (Government OSI Profile) for use by public bodies, and within GOSIP, the UN EDIFACT (Electronic Data Interchange for Administration, Commerce and Transport) protocol for NHS use. Health Level 7 (HL7) is widely used in the USA.

A *functional standard* and a *functional profile* have also to be adopted. The OSI (see above) provides a framework under which are collected over 150 standards for communications between computers. These standards are distributed between different levels – from standards at the level of the bare physical connections between machines to standards at a level which enables information and instruction to pass between computers. At each level an information system should conform to one of the OSI standards for that level, but each level has many possible standards (and some standards have variants. A functional profile states which standard an information system will adopt at each level. A functional standard is the functional profile recommended by or for an organisation.

The selection phase ends with a system purchase. Only now should the manager agree to meet any computer or information system salesmen. If this happens any sooner, before the manager is able to stipulate what requirements the suppliers must tender against, the hospital risks buying by default what it suits the supplier to sell. In selecting software, one should not overlook the availability of *public domain software* for many simpler uses (such as word-processing and communications). For complex information systems there are advantages in buying modular software, in which large programs are constructed in self-contained units which can be repaired or altered individually without disrupting an entire computer system. Many industry-standard software packages (e.g. LOTUS, dBASE) also give the user some scope to adapt the software to individual requirements. Chapter 11 considers the selection of hardware and software in more detail.

The *installation* phase ends with the handover of a working system to line managers. Taking delivery of the hardware and software is the least of the tasks involved. Depending on the case, other tasks may include rewiring the buildings (both for power and for datalinks), altering the telephone system, or even reconfiguring workplace layout. This work may extend outside the workplace, for instance if a hospital installs special link-lines to general practitioners (GPs). Staff training or retraining, or even recruitment of new staff, will often be necessary. So may training of other organisations, for instance of the GP fundholders or DHAs who may be linked to an NHS Trust by a new network. This may extend to patients themselves, if they are to use such technologies as *smart-card* patient records (see Chapter 8) or use automated self-monitoring equipment.

All this, however, pales besides the task of reorganising management and working practices around the new information system. The critical principle is to ensure that changes in workplace organisation are coordinated with information system changes; the ability of staff and managers to understand the new information, to see the practical implications and be able to implement them. Here one runs into all the complexity of implementing innovations and organisational change. Many texts explore the general principles (e.g. McCalman and Paton 1992) and Chapter 7 examines how these apply in the case of an NHS provider implementing a new information system, but two points deserve emphasis. One is the necessity of demonstrating benefits to the staff who will use the new system. Against the common presumption that employees are normally conservative towards workplace change, it should be noted that most employees do not oppose technical change *per se* but do, very rationally, oppose technical change which reduces their rewards from working, exposes their lack of competences or makes them redundant. The second point is that staff (and managers) need time to familiarise themselves with new information systems and unfamiliar, intimidating new information technologies. A system plan notes the long- and short-term priorities, task sequence, timescale and review points governing implementation of a new information system.

First use and problem identification consists of practically testing the hardware, then installing and checking the software (here the advantages of modular software in allowing piecemeal testing and rectification become evident). The main tasks are *prototyping* (developing experimental first versions of the hardware system and software), *debugging* (removing faults in the writing of the software by practical trial and error) and *compliance testing* (to ensure the information system, or parts of it, comply with buyer specifications). Standard approaches include *benchmark testing*, in which the time new software takes to run, its reliability and its demands on hardware and human operators are compared with an industry-standard 'benchmark' piece of software. This is also a testing phase for the supplier support. The experience of the London ambulance service underlines the necessity of 'double running' during this phase, with both old and new systems available until the new system has been proved workable, robust and reliable.

At this stage, rates of work are usually initially slower with a new automated information system than with the old (automated or manual) system until staff become confident, skilled and familiar with the new system, hence able to exploit all its capabilities. Alongside this are the tasks of dealing with the organisational implications of the new information, for instance the responses of doctors who for the first time find aspects of their clinical practice open to critical – and factually-based – scrutiny.

Routine running and problem resolution is an open-ended phase continuing for the whole life of the information system. Here, too, there is a 'make-or-buy' choice. In information system contexts *facilities management* means 'subcontracting an outside firm (or firms) to operate information systems on site', as (US) Kodak has subcontracted IBM to run its data centre, as many UK healthcare organisations now have. Such a contract may cover any of system maintenance, the initial inputting of data, and subsequent routine data maintenance and updating. This raises the question of whether outsider access to medically or commercially sensitive information is permissible (Burch and Grudnitski 1986: 474). Routine running and problem resolution depends more than might first appear on the quality of the system *documentation*: the instruction manuals, technical manuals, written standards, protocols, etc. and trouble-shooting guides which normally ought to be supplied with the hardware and software. It is often inevitable that these are voluminous but not (although common) that they are illegible, incomplete or unintelligible to anyone but the technical expert. The importance of ensuring daily (or more frequent) backup of data and other work cannot be overstated, especially when staff are new to automated information systems and liable to perceive backup as a chore and waste of disc space. A less frequent but equally necessary routine is *system audit*; checks to ensure that standards for coding, backing up and other routine working practices are being maintained and updated, and checks upon who is using the information produced by the system, and for what purposes.

Information system purposes formulated at the preselection stage are the criteria for system audit. This feedback loop brings us back to the question of the relation between information systems and management. The next four chapters examine this relationship at different levels within the NHS.

Chapter 2

INFORMATION MANAGEMENT AND TECHNOLOGY STRATEGY FOR HEALTHCARE ORGANISATIONS

Victor Peel

NHS Information management and technology strategy

Developing a supportive, affordable and achievable information and technology strategy for any large and complex organisation, particularly in health care, is exceptionally difficult. This chapter considers what the term 'strategy' might mean in this context, who is responsible for articulating this strategy, what an effective linkage between organisational goals and such a strategy might look like, what the key components of a local strategy are, and how one might start to implement it.

Until 1984 most NHS investment decisions on health information technology and most of the work on defining information requirements had been dealt with by the Department of Health and/or the RHAs, not locally. The largest proportion of information and IT investment had been on national research and for demonstration projects (e.g. the national Hospital Standard Systems Project), business management systems (e.g. regional payroll, supplies or personnel systems, Family Health Services Authority (FHSA) administration, or the national Standard Accounting System) or *ad hoc* individual projects, usually developed to stand alone and meet the needs of individual departments. Some were clinical (e.g. renal systems) but most were hospital administrative support systems (e.g. patient data systems). Very few information system developments were relevant to community-based or general practitioner services. There had been some earlier attempts to develop integrated information and IT strategies (e.g. at the London Hospital).

The technology implications of the Körner Reports (DHSS 1982) and the information implications of the Griffiths report (Department of Health 1983) led to the first DHSS commitment to recurrent annual investment in hospital information systems, including nursing and case-mix management information systems, of several hundred million pounds. By 1986 there was increasingly urgent need to integrate the planning of investment in such systems with the information requirements of clinical, administrative and managerial staff, if only to prevent considerable duplication of effort. The Department of Health hoped to minimise this waste by so defining the goals of such a strategy, its guiding principles and the specific actions to be taken at national, regional and local levels, as to produce a national information framework for local investment decisions on IT systems. But not until 1988 was there the first systematic attempt by the Department of Health in England to encourage, then require, formal, written strategies for each regional, district and other health authority. The Welsh NHS anticipated this need from the outset of its involvement with information management (Welsh Office 1990b).

In a national health service there are immense opportunities to research, plan, test, invest and train in a coordinated but decentralised way that cannot be done in more fragmented, local-service based health systems. The NHSME aspires to develop healthcare information and systems more quickly by following a nationwide but decentralised strategy than by leaving these decisions to the market or by having all investment controlled centrally. The practicability of achieving these benefits is, as yet, largely unproven. Nevertheless, it remains UK government policy that guiding principles for the wider and greater good must be complied with by each constituent NHS organisation. Its essential minimum requirements are that the principles underlying an information management and technology policy should be consistent with the wider UK health policy and strategies (see Chapter 1). NHS information systems must support defined clinical and other operational objectives, and positive steps must be taken to identify and realise their benefits. All information and IT projects over a threshold amount (in 1994, £1 million) should be subject to Treasury approval and each NHS organisation should have an information management and technology strategy explicitly related to its goals. That strategy should explicitly state what benefits are to be obtained from investment in information management and technology and how; in particular, what personal and organisational development is necessary to achieve this. Probity and value for money must be demonstrable at all times.

To these ends the national *Information Management and Technology Strategy* (NHSME-IMG 1992a) was published in December 1992, causing many NHS organisations to rethink their information policy and practice. The strategy aims to define a national infrastructure from information sharing and support for the development of local skills. It also aims to assist local choice in end-user systems through nationally funded development and exemplar projects; and to ensure value for money for local purchasers by minimising reinvention.

A UK national information infrastructure will support the sharing of information throughout the NHS. For this purpose, the information management and technology (IM&T) strategy advocates a set of linked policies. All information systems should be person-based, because care must be focused on the needs of individuals and integrated across the healthcare organisations with which they come into contact. If information is person-based, data need only be entered once and can be shared easily between organisations, minimising the data entry required. An NHS number will be used as the standard, unique personal identifier for each patient within all NHS systems. Until 1994, individuals were identified by a number of different codes, presenting a major barrier to integration of different data about the same person. The new NHS number is scheduled to be implemented throughout the NHS by 1995. Hitherto basic information about the same patient has often been held on separate FHSA, DHA, child health community and hospital systems. This duplication is wasteful and potentially inaccurate. A set of nationally linked NHS administrative registers will be created and shared by all local users. Whether and how this data can be linked with general practitioner and other (e.g. local authority) systems is under discussion.

There will be a strategy and system for NHS-wide data exchange. A networking policy will cover both voice and data communications. There has been significant expenditure in locally useful but nationally incompatible networks. Consequently, there will be national standards for machine-to-machine communications. Standards such as UN EDIFACT are required to achieve the required accuracy, speed and cost effectiveness in electronic communications. Since personal data will be communicated more quickly and widely, a national policy and framework is necessary to ensure confidentiality and security of person-based information.

For clinical purposes, a thesaurus will be compiled of coded clinical terms employed by doctors, nurses and therapists throughout the NHS. Read codes are being introduced through medical audit and resource management (see Chapter 9, pages 138–9). Soon many GP systems will also adopt the Read classifications and hospitals will move from ICD9 to ICD10 (International Classification of Diseases) (see Chapter 9). The thesaurus will also synchronise these changes.

All this demands implementation of programmes for training, education and development of local resources in support of information management and technology. A strategy for IM&T training and development, financed by the NHSME and run by the NHS Training Directorate (NHSTD) was established in 1991. These efforts must accompany organisational change, including that facilitated by information systems.

The most important justification for investment in healthcare systems will be their contribution to the quality and cost effectiveness of direct patient care. So information should focus on health and not merely the incidence of illness and the provision of treatment. Information systems must capture, analyse and report on data which demonstrate the progress of policies and programmes, such as *Health of the Nation* (Department of Health 1992), in achieving targets. Person-based health records enable the production of data about the health needs, lifestyle and morbidity profile of the local population. This is why individual patients' medical or clinical records should provide the primary building block for information systems development to support the delivery of high quality care to the individual.

Information systems must support the basic process of providing or commissioning high quality, cost-effective health services. The national IM&T strategy will focus on maximising purchasing power, minimising reinventions, and providing guidance to the supplier community. Increasing sophistication of systems will support a move to more complex and specific contracting, and bring about more effective monitoring of contracts and health interventions, or health gain (see Chapter 3). More accurate and compatible records of care facilitate clinical audit resource management activities.

As for the information systems themselves, data should be entered into NHS systems only once and then shared (within the limits of confidentiality) and validated on entry. Appropriate levels of security and confidentiality for healthcare information must be respected. Standards should allow the integration of software from different suppliers and allow software to run on a range of hardware platforms from different suppliers. Information systems should support clerical, management and organisational initiatives and management information should be produced wherever possible, as a by-product of clinical and other operational systems. All this must be accompanied by appropriate management development and training.

Together these principles are intended to provide for an integrated approach to the management of information and the development of computer systems and work processes. To this end NHSME intends actively to support exemplar projects.

Hospital healthcare is all about meeting the needs of patients. What are the most significant benefits that patients ought to receive as a result? Some of the clear improvements that patients will benefit from as the strategy is implemented include shorter waiting times because appointments are scheduled efficiently and more accurate diagnosis because records are known and tests are available; fewer overnight stays because clinical care is scheduled more efficiently, and less frustration because their records are available to carers without delay throughout the health service.

How will the strategy be realised? Among its objectives relating directly to hospital providers are that all trusts will develop an IM&T strategy identifying the range of information systems appropriate to its activities and the means of integrating them. It should also cover communications needs and the hospital's approach to joining the national infrastructure. All specialities should have systems to support medical audit, and all hospitals should have links with general practices. Generally, there is little experience in the NHS in preparing such documents. This brings us to the question of how to implement an NHS information system at a local level, in ways which both pursue these national strategies and reflect the local health organisation's own interests and imperatives.

Organisation-wide information strategy

This section explains how an information strategy is produced and how it relates to an NHS organisation's business plan. It also explains some connections between this information strategy and central information systems (IS) initiatives, such as the national IM&T strategy described in the previous section, then outlines some practical considerations in preparing a local IS and IT plan.

An organisation's information strategy is aimed at ensuring that its information systems and information technology are linked to and support its objectives, as Chapter 1 explained. Organisational change alters roles and responsibilities within an organisation and can also introduce new functions. NHS reforms are producing unusually wide-ranging and fundamental changes of this kind: the purchaser–provider split; new GP contracts and fundholding; the introduction of NHS Trusts and (in Scotland) agency services; resource management projects; and the consequent internal re-organisations within HAs and providers. In these conditions an NHS organisation's global purposes in drawing up an information strategy will include facilitating the operation of the internal market; monitoring NHS performance and management to achieve better resource use; improving the quality of patient care; encouraging the analysis of clinical activity; improving information on the health status of the population and monitoring it; and planning or providing healthcare to meet the population's needs. These exigences are best addressed by developing information systems in a structured way.

The main steps in deriving an information strategy from a business strategy in a healthcare organisation are to:

1 model the enterprise and its functions
2 chart the organisation and map the functions onto it
3 establish a hierarchy of goals
4 identify critical success factors for the whole organisation
5 break down broad organisational functions into specific tasks

6 identify the key information needed
7 choose the information systems and technologies required.

Business modelling is a useful technique for taking the first four steps. The technique is one of summarising the organisation's plans, goals, activities and structure in order to infer its high level information systems and data

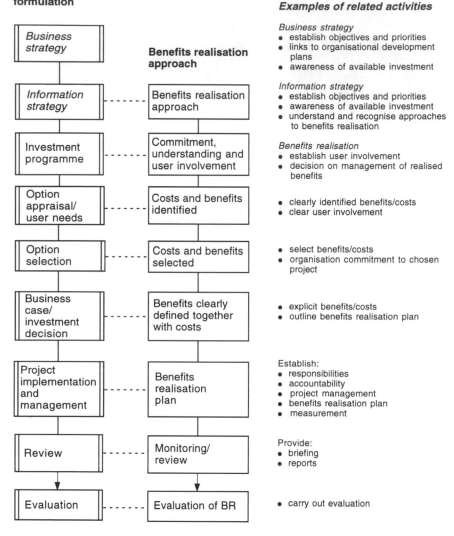

Information strategy formulation

Examples of related activities

Business strategy
- establish objectives and priorities
- links to organisational development plans
- awareness of available investment

Information strategy
- establish objectives and priorities
- awareness of available investment
- understand and recognise approaches to benefits realisation

Benefits realisation
- establish user involvement
- decision on management of realised benefits

- clearly identified benefits/costs
- clear user involvement

- select benefits/costs
- organisation commitment to chosen project

- explicit benefits/costs
- outline benefits realisation plan

Establish:
- responsibilities
- accountability
- project management
- benefits realisation plan
- measurement

Provide:
- briefing
- reports

- carry out evaluation

Flow (left column): Business strategy → Information strategy → Investment programme → Option appraisal/user needs → Option selection → Business case/investment decision → Project implementation and management → Review → Evaluation

Benefits realisation approach (middle column): Benefits realisation approach → Commitment, understanding and user involvement → Costs and benefits identified → Costs and benefits selected → Benefits clearly defined together with costs → Benefits realisation plan → Monitoring/review → Evaluation of BR

Figure 2.1   Information strategy and benefits realisation
Source: Benefits Realisation Advisory Group (1994)

requirements. It concentrates on reaching an understanding of an organisation's objectives and plans, thereby identifying the functions and data required to fulfil them. Its focus is on business functions, on analysing what the organisation plans to do and how it plans to do it rather than organisational structures or information technology. For example, a HA's functions would include health needs assessment, contract planning and placement, and contract management and monitoring (see Chapter 3). An agency's functions would include business planning, marketing, costing and monitoring services and quality standards; those of a healthcare provider include business planning, costing and pricing, contract negotiation, contract monitoring, capital charging, medical audit, activity recording and contract billing (see Chapters 5 and 12). Where these functions reside within the organisation is not a primary concern of an information strategy. Nevertheless, it is useful to consider how functions map back onto the organisational structure since this indicates where the information users are and highlights overlapping roles and responsibilities. All this helps define information system application areas by analysing the relationship between business functions and their information requirements. (Chapter 1 explains the concept of 'applications'.) The conclusions are then communicated to senior managers for them to verify (or correct), helping generate senior management commitment to the information strategy that follows. The process of preparing for an information strategy can be a means to promote discussion within the organisation about its priorities for information systems.

An information strategy is a strategy for both information systems and information technology. It is a formal plan for introducing, maintaining and supporting information systems and information technology in an organisation. Normally, an information strategy specifies:

1 The organisation's main objectives, functions and plans.
2 A benefits realisation analysis (see Chapter 1), explicitly linking the information strategy to the business model. The 'benefits' identified in the benefits realisation sections of the information strategy are the ways in which information systems and information technology are intended to contribute directly to the organisation's hierarchy of goals. Figure 2.1 shows how a benefits realisation approach frames the remainder of an information strategy.
3 The information needs corresponding to each function, and to the main tasks within each function. Table 2.1 illustrates what these might be for an NHS healthcare provider.
4 The consequent data requirements and sources. Whatever these are, the information strategy for any NHS organisation must (according to the national IM&T strategy) stipulate use of the NHS's Common Data Definitions. The organisation's information strategy should also identify means to simplify data collection (e.g. by collecting data from 'operational'

systems wherever possible) and to avoid duplicating data collection (e.g.
by linking information systems).

5 By comparing the organisation's information needs against current
systems, current objectives and the national IM&T strategy it will be
possible to assess how gaps in currently available information can best be
filled.

Table 2.1 Information requirements for an NHS
healthcare provider; an illustration

Integrated provision of care

*An initial list of functions to be satisfactory to those
participating in the care contract process*

---

 1 Complete tracking of events
 2 Accurate baseline clinical record
 3 Comprehensive events record
 4 Complete referrals record and consequences
 5 All requests for clinical/social services logged
 6 All reports for clinical/social services received
 7 Epidemiological data on 'local' services collected
 8 Prescribing and repeat prescribing analysis
 9 Clinical audit database
10 Shared care facility
11 Doctors office practice management functions
12 Health screening process facilities
13 Automatic summary of key events
14 (a) Cost/contract management function
     (b) Resource allocation information
     (c) Resource use information

An information strategy is above all a strategy and a plan for addressing
these information gaps through new or modified information systems and
information technology applications. The information and data requirements stated in the information strategy imply the logical architecture of the
information systems which will be created by implementing it. A logical
architecture is an overview of what applications (see Chapter 1) can be
delivered to users, how they will be delivered and how data can be managed
to support these applications. A physical architecture defines the technical
means of implementing the logical architecture. Translating logical into
physical architecture produces a range of evaluation criteria for choosing
between the physical options, taking into account the organisation's
environmental, technical, management and business circumstances. These

criteria will typically include assessments of how far the various information technology options:

1 fit into the organisation
2 are likely to have practical impact
3 carry risks
4 are technically feasible
5 have a favourable cost-benefit ratio
6 generate new staffing requirements.

In this way an information technology strategy flows from an organisation's wider information strategy. An IT strategy will normally specify:

1 existing information systems and technology
2 application requirements
3 technical support
4 what hardware and software will be procured, and how
5 communications strategy
6 consortium arrangements (if any)
7 staffing and training implications
8 IT audit and review arrangements
9 how the information systems will be managed
10 confidentiality and security requirements
11 a costed implementation timetable.

This implies an implementation programme which in turn requires funding. Where these requirements are similar to those of other trusts or Health Authorities it makes sense to consider bulk procurement and support arrangements. Common standards for hardware, software, communications and data definitions offer benefits in terms of data interchange and procurement policy, and an IT strategy should stipulate how far these are to be achieved.

A typical planning horizon for an information strategy would be three years with more detailed planning for year one of the cycle. The difference between a strategic and a tactical approach to information system development is more than a difference in length of planning period, as Table 2.2 summarises.

Methodologies offer a structured approach to the project of producing an information strategy and the corresponding information system plans, and implementing both (e.g. ETHICS, PRINCE, SSADM; see Chapter 1). A methodology usually comprises of a set of techniques and software tools to assist the project team such as project planning 'templates', business modelling software and data modelling software. Each methodology yields specified 'deliverables' from each phase of the project. Examples include application profiles for new systems or project implementation plans. Each methodology offers its own distinctive approach; its own list of the required

Table 2.2   Strategic and tactical approaches to information system planning

	Strategic	*Tactical*
Level of conduct	High management	Lower management
Regularity	Continuous irregular	Periodic fixed
Subjective values	Heavily weighted	Less weighted
Range of alternatives	Many	Few
Uncertainty	Considerable, more risk	Lower risk
Nature of problems	Unstructured, one-off	Structured repetitive
Information needs	Much external, future	Less internal, historical
Time horizons	Longer	Shorter
Completeness	Whole organisation	Sub-organisations
Detail	Broad	Narrow
Personnel involved	Top management, few	Many
Ease of evaluation	Difficult	Easier
Objectives, policies, strategies	New	Familiar
Point of view	Corporate	Functional

tasks, their logical sequence and timescale. Its approach will also specify the types of documentation needed at each stage and imply specific project management processes and lines of communications within the organisation.

Nevertheless, most methodologies take a fundamentally common approach to putting together an information strategy. The basic tasks they cover involve:

1 defining what information the organisation needs
2 assessing how well current arrangements meet that need
3 describing the hardware, software, organisational and people-related projects that need to be initiated to address the gaps between information need and provision
4 defining priorities, timescales and costed resource requirements for implementing the strategy programme.

Working methods used to achieve these basic tasks typically include workshops, small group discussions, interviews, presentations and desk research. A methodology usually includes examples of documentation. These are useful both as a reminder of what needs to be covered in a particular stage and as a means of documenting findings. Examples of methodology documentation include checklists (useful when interviewing and for documenting existing information systems), matrices (mapping information needs against the organisation's functions), questionnaires (guidance for interviews), forms (documentation of existing systems, application profiles, project descriptions) and diagrams (e.g. of data models, application models, hardware and communications linkages).

There are considerable benefits in using a structured methodology. These include clear guidance on what tasks are required and their sequence. By providing a set of guidelines and checklists a methodology can also suggest how each task in the project should be handled and documented. A structured approach gives rigour, direction and productivity to the process of deciding the information strategy and yields managerial products in a usable format. It offers a ready-formed documentation system, and external training and support in using the better-established methodologies is available. A structured methodology is a mechanism for involving senior staff in producing the information strategy and improving dialogue between information system users and strategists. The information strategy document itself can help inform staff on what initiatives apply to their area of the organisation and over what timescale.

For a methodology to work in practice it needs to cover the process of information system development comprehensively through to post-installation review, and to be usable by staff of varying abilities. It must aid project planning by suggesting project phases and incorporate useful tools and techniques at appropriate stages in the project. Given limitations on timescales and resources, and the fact that it needs to cope with both large and small projects, the methodology must also be flexibly adaptable to suit project requirements. A useful concept in tailoring a chosen methodology to a particular project requirement is that of 'route mapping'. Not all steps within a methodology will always be used for a given strategy. Route mapping allows the project team to select the most appropriate route through the methodology to suit the needs of the project. By route mapping a path through the methodology the project team can focus on the priorities for the study and be clear as to those aspects of the methodology that they are skipping over for practical reasons. Throughout the project of devising an information strategy a focus on robust conclusions and practical implementation are prerequisites for success.

Factors determining the success of projects to decide an information strategy, plan an information system or install new information technology relate more to people than to systems, technology or methodology. The process by which the information strategy is produced is as important as its content in this respect. Success factors include:

1 Achieving staff ownership of the information strategy through involving them in formulating it (see also Chapter 7).
2 Having a suitable mixture of project skills (IS skills, IT skills, user views, management skill); consider getting external help, but support and advice, not the delivery of whole strategies or systems.
3 Good communications within the organisation, involving the right people.
4 Realistic budgets and timescale – slow down if necessary.
5 Identifying and resolving 'issues'.

6 The support of (but not excessive reliance on) a methodology.
7 Relating the local project to national strategic priorities and frameworks.
8 Looking for ways of improving use of existing information and systems.
9 Establishing the infrastructure required to implement the strategy.
10 Incorporating information strategy and planning into the general management of the organisation.

Structured methodologies for producing information strategies can provide benefits if applied sensitively and flexibly. They should inform and support the planning process, not dictate it. Information strategy and information system planning is not a theoretical exercise but about people, how they do their jobs, and how information technology can help them.

Chapter 3

PURCHASER INFORMATION SYSTEMS

Rod Sheaff

Existing purchaser information systems

A large part of the defence of the NHS reforms is the suggestion that the NHS internal market will be a managed market. This, it is argued, will preserve the principle of free access to healthcare and the provision of healthcare on the basis of needs (Department of Health 1989a) and is what differentiates the NHS reforms from a straightforward privatisation. Recent policy statements emphasise that this will require a strengthening of purchasers' roles in the internal market (Bottomley 1993; Malwhinney 1992). These roles largely consist of the collection, analysis and managerial use of information. What information purchasers require for their new roles, the next section examines. This section starts by reviewing what their current information systems can do.

Recent policy gives the role of NHS purchasers as:

> assessing the health needs of their local populations and purchasing the services most appropriate to those needs from a range of providers . . . ensuring a better balance between hospital and community health services and primary care services. (Department of Health 1993b: 1)

To this the Department of Health adds 'concentrating scarce resources (e.g. in public health and information management) and maximising management cost savings' (Department of Health 1993b: 12).

All this is done through the healthcare purchasing cycle. Setting aside minor differences in how different sources label them, the healthcare purchasing cycle incorporates the following steps (or the equivalent):

1 health profiling
2 projecting health profiles for the contract period
3 identifying what morbidities in this projected health profile are preventable or treatable
4 determining best achievable health gain for each constituent of the health profile
5 formulating local health gain targets
6 costing these targets
7 allocating cash
8 provider selection
9 letting and monitoring service contracts.

Steps 1 to 5 make what might be called the 'purchaser-led' needs assessment, using demographic data and epidemiological knowledge. The corresponding user-led needs assessment is added as part of step 8, using adaptations of marketing information systems. Feedback from step 9 informs (or should do) the next iteration of steps 1 to 7. One should note that this is a normative model. Most DHAs and consortia actually derive their purchasing policies by adjusting past purchasing patterns at the margins, not in the zero-based approach implied above (Redmayne et al. 1993). But supposing they did follow the above cycle, what information systems can purchasers currently call upon?

Such a cycle has been used to structure the Public Health Information Specification (PHIS), itself part of the Developing Information Systems for Purchasers (DISP) project (Wain and Holton 1993). DISP is intended to become the kernel of purchaser information systems. The DISP Health Information Workstation (HIW) combines data from Office of Population Consensus and Surveys (OPCS) censuses and population projections, the Public Health Common Data Set, Health Service Indicators, Vital Statistics, a population health register, a record of health-related events, Regional activity and deaths data. The Public Health Data Set includes data on causes of death overall, mortality due to the commoner types of cancer and cardio-thoracic conditions, suicide, accidents, stillbirth and perinatal death; and low birthweight data. Until NHS Administration Registers are available, FHSA registers will be used instead. The Welsh Population Health Summary System is to combine such an all-Wales register with a personal health summary for each person, noting their permanent medical characteristics (e.g. allergies), medical episodes and current medical problems (Goldberg et al. 1993).

DISP also contains a contract and invoice management system based on per-patient episodes and provider data. A corollary will be for purchasers to devise standard codes for purchasing organisations (including GP fundholders), contracts, service type (to distinguish outpatients from day-patients from inpatients, and so on) and the actual service provided. DISP is being developed from the DISS prototypes piloted at Cambridge, Leeds, Sheffield and Walsall in 1990–91. NHSME plans to extend DISP by using the new NHS number in the Administrative Register, and adding data on GP fundholders, primary care, community care and *Health of the Nation* indicators, besides a commercial products review and a thesaurus of clinical terms and coding (based on Read codes; see Chapter 9). NHSME also plan to strengthen the system's ability to network with the information systems of other agencies, particularly local authorities' (NHSME-IMG 1993b).

Commercial systems are now becoming available both for service contracting purposes and to build on the Sheffield project. WHO (Europe) is developing a health indicators mapping system with the obvious advantage of assisting international comparisons. Richards (1993: 245–66) records three local geographic systems. Health profiles are published at UK level (Department of Health, annually) but they do not exhaust the content noted above, neither are they disaggregated to DHA or locality level; locality profiling is still at an early stage of automation as part of DISP (Wain 1993 gives an example). Local population profiles will also be necessary for funding purchasers by capitation from 1993–4 (Malin 1992; NHSME 1993c). OPCS data shows the frequency of complaints causing disability (OPCS 1988). *Local Voices* emphasises the importance of collecting information on local consumers' perceptions of NHS services and their preference for service developments but gives only cursory guidance on the information systems aspect of this (NHSME 1992c).

For calculating achievable health gain and monitoring progress towards it the new outcome indicator database at the Nuffield Centre, Leeds is potentially an important development, although the database will initially concentrate on indicators for acute care. The NHSME has funded publication of these indicators. For intersectoral activity some indicators are already in *Health for All 2000* and NHSME is elaborating those required for monitoring *Health of the Nation*. To analyse the social mix of local populations the Jarman Underprivileged Area Score became available from the 1989–90 HSI package but only at DHA or FHSA level and calculated from 1981 OPCS census data (the similar Department of Employment Social Index became available one year earlier). NHS organisations' access to library and databases remains generally underdeveloped (McDougall and Brittain 1992: 23).

There are moves besides DISP towards strengthening information systems for provider selection and resource allocation. For instance the Priority system uses cost-per-QALY (quality-adjusted life year) data for some 200 interventions, population preference weightings and indicators of 'local equity judgements' to rank purchasing options. It analyses the results by group and subgroup, also showing for incremental changes and sensitivity analysis. One Scottish implementation uses data covering some 70 per cent of the Scots population (Hudson 1993; Twaddle 1993). The Health Promotion Authority Wales and University College Wales are developing a database for Health Authorities on health promotion resources, contacts and statistics (Cook 1992). NHSME Purchaser Marketplace Forum meetings and other networks are already developing to share qualitative 'market intelligence'. A more ambitious, but also a younger, project is the Welsh Benchmarking Centre, which aims to collect current data on 'best practice' in all main areas of clinical work.

Provider selection requires a means of comparing providers' performance in terms of cost and workload in a way that standardises the differences in case mix between the different providers. In the US health system DRGs were developed for this purpose (see Chapters 9 and 12). English experiments with DRG (Diagnostic Related Group)-based case combines mix systems began in 18 sites in 1986 for purposes which were not then entirely clear (Newman and Jenkins 1991: 5–8, 26–7; see Chapter 9). The NHS will adopt Health Resource Groups, a derivative of DRGs by 1994. APGs (Ambulatory Patient Groups) are not yet officially being developed in the UK although commercial development is under way. A few NHS documents almost recognise that comparisons of the health gain achieved by different providers also require standardisation for case mix (cf. Bullas 1989: 15):

> Care profiles would eventually contain expected outcome measures and ranges of values of such measures for the groups. A number of studies and experiments in the use of outcome measures are taking place, the results of which will provide further details. (Bullas 1989: 11)

Current UK case mix systems can provide data necessary for such comparisons but do not yet actually perform the analysis. Even the use of HRGs (health resource groups) is not yet (1994) mandatory (NHSME 1992f). Meanwhile as a surrogate for direct comparisons of quality, protocols of acceptable clinical procedures for routine treatment plans are being developed in some parts of the NHS (e.g. NHSME 1991b). The nearest (but not very near) equivalent UK data to the US comparisons of provider safety and cost are the annual CEPOD (Confidential Enquiry on Maternal Deaths) Parliamentary Commissioner and Community Health Council (CHC) reports, and the limited publicly available data on unplanned readmissions, hospital-acquired infections, waiting lists and Patients' Charter standards. Comparative data on provider outcomes and quality is not envisaged in 'organisational audit' nor in CEPOD (except in anonymised summary annual reports).

DISP will provide much of the data necessary for routine administration of service contracts (universal use of a national patient, GP and purchaser identifiers, besides clinical coding) if it develops as anticipated. Experiments have taken place in networking such information using OSI principles (see Chapter 1) as a preliminary to a national NHS network. NSHME is developing Contract Minimum Data Sets and Data Interchange Standards for them, to use EDIFACT (Electronic Data Interchange for Administration,

Commerce and Transport) protocols (EL(92)34, 28 May 1992). It is also considering minimum standards for all prescribing and dispensing machines (McDougall and Brittain 1992: 32). The NHS Coding and Classification Centre is adopting Read coding, with various modifications including mapping onto ICD9 and OPCS codes, and undertaking a clinical terms project, to standardise codes, data and terminology for all the above purposes. More immediately, NHSME proposes to publish 'league tables' on hospital waiting times and cancelled operations (*The Guardian* 7 December 1993). Purchaser and provider efficiency and activity levels are measured by a formula which combines crude activity data for five broad categories of activity, weighted by their share in the previous financial year's expenditure, then compares the proportionate change with the change in real-terms expenditure (NHSME 1993c). It has been criticised for re-warding the use of hospital (especially outpatient) services (Evans 1993). It is also fallacious because average total cost is no index of efficiency (Neumann *et al.* 1992: 9). DHAs are now having also to collect summary capital charging data and transmit them via RHAs to the NHSME (NHSME 1992g).

DISP and HIW are oriented primarily towards managing service contracts for secondary care. Yet administration of preventive health services depends even more obviously on complete and reliable information systems (e.g. for call and recall systems such as those for breast screening. Chapter 4 outlines the current state of FHSA information systems for managing general practice and other primary care services.

Information systems for supporting health promotion are still more fragmentary. This is particularly damaging because intersectoral activity works largely by publicising health data to support health education, social marketing, anti-marketing and political lobbying. Health data are the main working medium for influencing public behaviours and political decisions. The Big Kill and the Smee Report illustrate this. The Big Kill was a publicity campaign in which NHS staff calculated numbers of smoking-related deaths, apportioned these to hospital bed occupancy, then allocated bed occupancy because of smoking related disease to each parliamentary constituency, local authority and Health Authority. Information in this form was ready-made for presenting to MPs, pressure-groups and the press. The Smee report meta-analyses many-country evidence about the effects of advertising on total tobacco consumption, showing a small but significant correlation (Smee 1992). These findings made it harder for the UK government to oppose proposed EC smoking controls. Both cases illustrate what impact somewhat dry, obscure data can have when analysed and presented to expose causes of preventable ill-health and to connect them with the interests of those able to take action (e.g. by legislation, product redesign). Unfortunately, these two cases are exceptional, not routine, instances of the NHS and Department of Health using information to promote health.

Despite what has been done in developing purchaser information systems, the outstanding information demands posed by the purchasers' new roles in the internal market remain formidable. The next task is to consider what these demands are.

New information requirements for purchasing

Doubtless governments will continue to use healthcare purchasing to implement wider health policies such as public expenditure control, the Citizen's Charter and waiting list management. Nevertheless, NHS purchasers' *raison d'etre* is to maximise population health status (in practice, within budget). Within this, needs assessment generates the criteria for making 'rationing' decisions and for selecting service providers. The main task for purchaser information systems in future will therefore be to enable NHS purchasers do this more comprehensively and defensibly, using the results to manage the purchasing cycle noted in the previous section.

In descending order of health impact (and increasing order of NHS spending) three types of need assessment are necessary for purchasing purposes. From a profile of its healthy population a purchaser can assess needs for intersectoral health promotion and preventive health care. WHO describes intersectoral activity as:

> Linkages . . . with other sectors that control and influence factors that determine health – agriculture, food and nutrition, education and information, environment and physical infrastructure. The health sector should cooperate in the management of these factors for the promotion of health.   (WHO 1986: 123)

A second profile is of the population who do not enjoy full health, but whose condition is comparatively stable so that they need long-term care rather than acute health services. From this profile the needs for community care and social care, and the remaining long-term institutional care, and long-term maintenance care services (e.g. for the chronically sick such as diabetics) can be assessed. This leaves, thirdly, the profile of ill populations requiring acute GP and hospital services.

Each profile comprises data on a population's size and geographic distribution. It identifies the elderly, disabled and chronically ill populations, morbidity and mortality patterns, and their size and distribution by age, sex and locality. The types and sizes of these categories indicate the main care groups, defined sometimes by types of disease, sometimes by the type of intervention. Sometimes they coincide with a clinical speciality (e.g. for childbirth), sometimes not (e.g. for cancers). To assess the population's needs for health services over the contract period, local data on the main factors affecting population health status are necessary. These data would ordinarily include:

1 Social mix (class mix, occupation or unemployment, dependency ratio, ethnicity, and incomes; a powerful predictor of life expectancy (Doyal and Gough 1991: 278)).
2 Education, especially literacy, and housing.
3 Age-sex mix.
4 Physical environment (e.g. patterns of pollution, radioactivity levels).
5 Occupational hazards.
6 Health behaviours (smoking, nutrition, tourism, etc.).
7 Patterns of fertility and reproductive behaviour.

Health profiles have to be formulated in the medium of health status indicators, although at present (1994) these are only incompletely and imperfectly available. (Outcome indicators indicate changes in health status indicators attributable to health service interventions.) The profile should also include health service utilisation patterns, including use of health services outside the purchaser's territory and of health services not financed by the NHS (Pickin and St Leger 1993 suggest one way of doing this). Where, but only where, there is scientific evidence of the efficacy of health care, utilisation data can be used as proxies for health status data (e.g. for immunisation).

The next information task is to identify what impact health services can have on the morbidity, mortality and disability catalogued in the health profile. A preliminary calculation is how these will change over the contract (or in non-market systems, planning) period. The projected health profile assesses for the contract period what deaths, morbidity and disability it is necessary to prevent or remedy in the local population. Purchaser information systems might tackle this in two ways. A marginal approach would be to project the health profile on the assumption that health service purchasing, and the impact of these services, continues unaltered. This gives a comparitor against which the marginal health gains of alternative purchasing patterns can be compared (see below). A zero-based approach would be to project the health profile that would result if no health services were purchased at all, so as to identify the total health gains offered by different purchasing patterns. Automating either projection is not difficult; the difficulty lies in getting the data to project.

Given the projected health profile, it is then necessary to identify which deaths, morbidity and disabilities health services can prevent or treat. *Health For All 2000* is a reminder that fewer causes of ill-health are completely uninfluencable by purchasers than an orientation purely towards providing institutional services for patients might suggest. Supposing that the data collection problems and the lack of health status indicators were soluble, the main information problem here would lie in assembling and applying existing clinical and epidemiological knowledge about what causes of death, morbidity and disability are preventable and treatable, and to what degree. This requires purchaser information system links to research databases. Which health status indicators are sensitive to the effects of health service intervention, is an under-researched question (Martini et al. 1977). To fill the gaps requires a large amount of primary research. By showing which causes of death, morbidity and disability in the health profile are not yet amenable to prevention or effective treatment this analysis incidentally assesses needs for health service research and development.

For the ill-health that can be prevented or treated, it is next necessary to quantify the achievable health gain for each care group by discovering what interventions are available, which are most effective in clinical terms, and what effects they have. Insofar as it is known, this information can be obtained either from published research or from expert opinion or both. What health gain can be achieved for each sub-population is obviously contingent upon the current state of preventive and clinical technologies.

The Strategic Intent and Direction for the NHS in Wales (SID) includes protocols on the efficacy of clinical interventions and shows ways to derive service targets from them, initially for 10 health gain areas: cancers; cardiovascular disease; maternal and early child health; physical disability and discomfort; respiratory disease; injuries; mental handicap, illness and distress; emotional health and relations; environment; and lifestyle (Welsh Office, NHS Directorate 1990a). The method applies to any care group where suitable research findings exist. This demands, Welsh experience shows, a national or international centre to generate protocols through a critical scrutiny of clinical and epidemiological research. Purchasers' information systems have to be networked either to such a centre or directly to the clinical and epidemiological research databases, should purchasers prefer to write their own protocols.

On this basis, purchasers can formulate local health gain targets. Local formulation may be necessary for two reasons. Available providers may simply lack the 'best practice' providers' expertise or infrastructure (e.g. if the 'best practice' is abroad). More importantly, the health gain from 'best practice' in the settings from which research publications report may partly reflect the operation of 'confounding factors' besides the 'best practice' itself. The confounding factors have themselves to be quantified empirically in each case but commonly they will include the patients' age, sex and class mix, how patients were selected to receive the treatments which have been evaluated, and their health status at the start of the treatment (Inglis 1983). When the confounding factors can be quantified, local health gain targets should be standardised for local pecularities in these factors. (The health profile should note them.) To illustrate; in Britain the prevalence of smoking varies by social class. A purchaser serving a population with a high proportion of social classes 1 and 2 can realistically set providers of health promotion services a lower target level for numbers of young smokers than a purchaser for a similarly sized population with a high proportion of classes 4 and 5 could. These calculations too are easily automated provided research and local health profile data are available. Throughout these steps health status indicators remain the medium in which targets are formulated.

To make purchasing decisions it is necessary to cost the local health gain targets. An advantage in basing health gain targets on researched 'best practice' is that this also gives an approximation of what resources will be required. ('Approximation', because local providers may require different resources to implement 'best practice'.) Given providers' prices, a purchaser information system that had completed the preceding stages could now demonstrate what resources are necessary and sufficient, under present conditions and technologies, to meet current local population needs for health services (as opposed to their health needs – identified at step two). While prevention is normally better than cure in maximising health gain, preventive programmes take decades to bear fruit. There remain those whose health was already compromised before prevention became available and those suffering from as yet unpreventable illness. Costing based on targets derived from best practice and the projected health profile will for many years include 'double running' costs of running large-scale curative alongside preventive care for many groups of patients (e.g. cardiological patients). So the total resource required is likely to be large and might (but only 'might'; the point is not proved) grow continuously in future. It is certainly not infinite, as some suggest (Bottomley 1992); but probably will exceed the purchaser's budget.

Rationing decisions that convert assessments of needs for health services into a purchasing programme are then the seventh step; a matter of deciding whose healthcare needs not to meet. Information systems containing the above data could also make preliminary rankings of possible purchasing patterns, assuming the decision rule of always maximising health gain (partly because currently UK health policy requires this, but more importantly because of the intuitive plausibility of the idea). In logic, the ranking would proceed through the following steps. A preliminary would be to triage out purchases which:

1 Are iatrogenic or produce no nett health gain; ECT is arguably an example. A stronger interpretation would be to exclude all procedures lacking evaluative evidence of health gain. (Cochrane 1972 explained what this evidence would be, and for how many standard procedures it is absent.).
2 Are technically efficacious but give little or no health gain, such as minor cosmetic surgery or (more controversially) assisted reproduction.
3 Substitute models of care, or other providers, can replace at greater health gain, lower cost or both.

This leaves the harder question of how to prioritise among the remaining, unequivocally health-gain producing services.

Since health status depends largely on factors in the non-health sectors, information systems that evaluated locally achievable health gain would implicitly quantify what resources to allocate to health services and what to preventive work to maximise health gain. In descending order of likely health impact the other strategies for managing scarcity are: technological improvements in health service productivity; lobbying for greater resourcing; sharpening provider incentives; reallocating between services; and verbally defining demands away as not 'real health needs' (Sheaff and Peel 1993: 1.3). The effect of simply defining certain demands away is easily modelled from existing data but deciding what information is necessary to identify a health gain maximising allocation between the remaining strategies is a complex matter. One difficulty lies in making factual assumptions and predictions about the health impact of each set of strategies. They would presumably have to be generated from comparative and historical research at national or international level. In practice purchaser information systems would depend heavily on exploiting access to the appropriate sources of secondary research.

All this presupposes that the idea of 'maximising health gain' is unproblematic; an oversimplification. It brings us to the inherent limits of purchaser information systems. They cannot directly determine which aspects of purchasing decisions are properly a matter for expert (professional) decisions through technical (including clinical) evaluation, and which are properly decided by consumer preference. In a recent experiment, healthcare purchasers from the state of Oregon collected citizens' opinions about which healthcare procedures it was most desirable to purchase from Federally supported State budgets. These opinions were used to rank the list of available healthcare procedures. The purchaser then proposed to buy as many of the highest ranked procedures as were demanded, and so on down the list until the budget ran out (which happened about three-quarters of the way down the list). The damaging objection to the Oregon experiment lies here, not (primarily) in the alleged crudity of the consumer research or information systems used. The most sophisticated information system cannot redeem outcome indicators which are inherently biased in favour of some care groups, logically defective, or incorporate a fallacy. Harris' (1985) critique of QALYs illustrates some of the problems. Such indicators vitiate the information systems using them. Neither can information systems alone answer questions about which services ought to be provided – or prohibited – as a matter of principle (whether of rights, duties, social solidarity, or basic individual needs). These are matters for healthcare ethics and law. The most an information system can do is link the purchaser with relevant literature databases.

One way NHS purchasers can influence the internal market is by encouraging new providers to enter the market, increasing purchasers' bargaining power. Another is to support new models of care such as 'hospital at home'. Purchaser information systems would facilitate this if they had access to national or international registers of providers. If provider listing on the database depended on accreditation, licensing or verification of the provider's likely financial viability during a standard contract period, this would be a ready-made form of provider screening. Subscription databases on companies' financial state already operate in other sectors of the UK economy. Healthcare provider selection is an obvious candidate for a centralised, on-line provider database, perhaps similar to a selective Institute of Health Services Management (IHSM) *Yearbook* (IHSM, annually).

Price and quality are the two main criteria for selecting among providers (when budgets are cash limited, per-patient prices determine what volume of patients can be treated). United States experience suggests public purchasers can use price policy to influence healthcare market development by adjusting the comparative commercial attractiveness of different types of health service. An example is ProPAC's support during 1992 for 'swing beds' (ProPAC 1991; this is the US term for community hospital beds that can 'swing' between acute and long-term use). A UK equivalent would be premium pricing for, say, community care or day surgery. In a buyer's market this use of price policy is also available to GP fundholders. Early experience suggests that using price policy to influence service quality may be a more attractive use of pricing policy to GP fundholders than using price negotiations simply to contain costs (Glennerster *et al.* 1992). To compare providers' offer prices on a cost-per-treatment basis for block or cost and volume contracts, the offer prices must be standardised for case mix. Purchaser information systems must therefore analyse case mix using a national or international system (see Chapter 9). This is an argument against adopting non-standard grouping systems (such as the New York or Yale variants of DRGs) without some compensating benefit.

Debates about case mix systems usually assume that patient episodes, or bundles of them, are the commodity unit bought and sold. However, the development of outcome indicators, and the means of analysing health gain attributable to health services (see above) offers the technical possibility of moving away from event-based pricing towards benefit pricing: the purchaser paying for achievable health gain. In some specialities this prospect is not so distant as it sounds; the MNTK eye hospitals in St Petersburg have already been paid according to whether a forecast improvement in vision is achieved, or whether (in some contracts with employers) the patient can return to work. Automated testing systems and computer-aided diagnosis and prognosis (with and without treatment) reduce the scope for clinicians to estimate achievable vision gain too conservatively. Such systems require a combination of automated clinical records, expert clinical systems, and a database of past clinical outcomes.

Providers can be selected on two types of quality criteria: technical criteria and consumers' preference. To compare providers' performance technically, on outcome, would both initiate a database of suitable outcome indicators and data on alternate providers' performance against these indicators. A United States answer to both tasks is to establish a nationally Uniform Clinical Data Set (UCDS) to automate peer review (clinical audit) and produce a detailed, patient-level database which can also be used epidemiologically (ProPAC 1991: 51). Large commercial databases of this kind already exist and public ones in some States. In Philadelphia, for instance, *Hospital Effectiveness Reports* are published annually comparing named hospitals on patient numbers, their condition on admission, death rates, stay and price, comparing some of these variables with statistically expected levels (Pennsylvania Health Care Cost Containment Council, annually). Similar surveys have been made in Cincinnati although the results are not published. The comparative data are standardised for severity on patient admission. United States insurers run databases on negligence cases and BUPA in the United Kingdom has an extensive follow-up database but these are not published either.

Outcome comparisons of providers would have to standardise for case mix. Existing case mix measures (DRGs and HJRGs in particular) group patients whose care costs approximately equal amounts, because the purpose of the measures is to manage costs. Analogously, to manage outcomes by comparing providers requires patients to be grouped by approximate equality of attainable health gain. Such groupings are likely to differ from the isoresource groupings. So purchasers require a dual case mix system; one system for cost comparisons, one for 'real' (health gain) comparisons. Besides standardising for case mix, a comparison of different providers' contribution to health gain should also standardise for other exogenous influences on the health gain of different providers' patients – above all the class mix of the different patient populations.

To select among providers on grounds of consumer preference requires a dual marketing information system. Assessing public preferences demands behavioural information on referral patterns (particularly cross-boundary flows, ECRs (extra contractual referrals) and the use of private health services). Unless there are extenuating epidemiological circumstances, these are signs of what patients and GPs regard as inadequate service contracting. From data on referral sources it is possible to map the existing 'natural' patient flows and catchments for existing providers, suggesting which patient groups (by locality) are likely to be affected by switching patient flow to or from a particular provider. Commercial software for this is already available. Information on consumer attitudes and opinions can be collected by the usual market research methods. The best known (if not always the most suitable) is the questionnaire. This part of a purchaser information system demands qualitative (here, interpretive) as much quantitative information. For NHS purchasing purposes the term 'consumer' has to be taken to include GPs and informal carers (as proxy for patient's informed judgement) besides patients themselves.

The choice of criteria for provider selection also lies beyond the scope of information systems. One way to maximise the health gain for a given budget would be to list the providers in descending order of health gain-to-price ratio, then buy from these providers in descending order until either the budget or the need for that type of healthcare was exhausted. A special case is to offer providers a standard price for a service contract then select those offering the highest service quality. Conversely, a purchaser can insist providers satisfy minimum quality standards then select the lowest price (hence maximum volume for a given budget). Purchaser information systems can furnish the data and carry out the ranking calculations but not make the policy decision about how to judge the competition.

The last step in the purchasing cycle is to let, administer and monitor service contracts. Information systems can support this in four ways. First, comparing providers' capacity and purchasers' demand for each service indicates whether the purchaser is likely to achieve its purchasing targets and anticipates access problems (e.g. likelihood of waiting lists accumulating). Secondly, it indicates whether the purchaser confronts a buyer's or a seller's market. Information can be used to inform negotiations with providers in much the same ways the next section illustrates from the provider side. Thirdly, informed preference and information can be a source of pressure on providers. An illustration is West Midlands RHA's publication, in September 1993, of per-consultant waiting times for non-urgent hospital treatment. Fourthly, purchasers have an interest in agreeing what monitoring data feedback is included in the price of a service contract. The choice of monitoring indicators is critical because it is tantamount to the choice of provider incentives. Cornwall HA periodically monitors some long-stay residential care using outcome indicators; this is in principle the optimum monitoring indicator and incentive.

Monitoring service contract compliance requires basic information on who is being treated, where and for what. A prudent purchaser will collect and verify information on what services have been provided before paying the provider (Claydon 1992). Such information is at present only available patchily to NHS purchasers although the work can be automated by networking hospital, GP fundholder, DHA and FHSA information systems, as can the actual payment. Automating medical data interchange and analysis demands common (ideally, international) communications carrier standards, data standards, codes (Benson 1991: 3, 81, 83, 87), medical nomenclature and classifications.

Purchasers are also charged with publicising locally what services have been contracted for, what consumers can reasonably expect from providers (and what to do if they do not get it) and why certain services (e.g. sterilisation reversal, assisted conception) are not available. An informational system on the above lines also generates the content of these messages; why the purchasing organisation purchases what it purchases. Deciding how to formulate the message, which target audiences to address it to, and by which media requires opinion survey data (maybe as little as annually) and smaller-scale market research for pilot-testing proposed publicity messages and materials. Much of it can be bought from specialist firms (e.g. Gallup, MORI) and in some places (e.g. Bradford) this has been done as a joint DHA-FHSA project (Wagner 1993).

The complexity, size and timescale of these informational tasks are large. Meanwhile, for patients the provision of healthcare starts (and in the great majority of cases finishes) in primary and community health services. An overview of provider information systems therefore begins there.

Chapter 4

PRIMARY HEALTHCARE AND GENERAL PRACTICE

Chris Mackintosh and Gina Shakespeare

FHSA information systems: the current position

DHA information systems support the purchasing of secondary care. Their equivalent in respect of general practitioners are FHSA information systems. The computerisation of Family Practitioner Committees (FPCs – the immediate ancestor of the FHSAs) is a rare example of a highly centralised NHS information technology investment programme, reflecting the direct management of FPCs by the Department of Health until the NHS and Community Care Act 1990. Until the early 1990s few FPCs had employed management information specialists. Not only was the information technology centrally prescribed, the software which operated was a national system, developed and supported by the FHS Computer Unit at Exeter with support teams based around the country. The main purposes of this system were to allow the FPC to maintain an accurate patient database, to support payments to family practitioners, to facilitate the transfer of medical records and to undertake the administration of screening programmes on behalf of DHAs. It was therefore an operational rather than a management information system.

In 1987 the government published the white paper, *Promoting Better Health* (DHSS 1987), aimed at changing the emphasis in Family Practitioner Services towards disease prevention and health promotion, and away from reactive care. Another key policy was the enhancement of accountability of general medical practitioners in particular. Previously, general practitioners were perceived to operate almost entirely autonomously. FPCs, concerned mainly with the 'pay and rations' functions of general practice, had been expected to plan and manage family practitioner services since the mid 1980s. They were neither equipped nor resourced to do this. In the wake of *Promoting Better Health* FPCs' powers were significantly enhanced as the first new contract for general medical practice in 30 years was negotiated between the Department of Health and the General Medical Services Committee (Department of Health, 1989c). The scene was set for FHSAs (the form in which FPCs were reorganised) to exercise increased control over general medical services via the new contract and with enhanced powers, notably control over the deployment of cash limited budgets for reimbursement of practice staffing and premises costs.

With *Working for Patients* (Department of Health 1989a) further changes were made. FHSAs became accountable to RHAs. Other changes included: a scheme to monitor and account for expenditure on drugs prescribed by GPs (Department of Health 1990e); the introduction of medical audit in general practice; FHSA general managers were appointed and management arrangements generally revised and upgraded. Of all the changes related to primary care brought about by *Working for Patients* particular emphasis was placed on the introduction of GP fundholding. The role which GPs could play by becoming the purchasers of specified hospital (and later community) services was pivotal to the NHS reforms and received enormous political and managerial attention. Parallels were drawn between the FHSA's 'new' role as a commissioner of primary care services from independent contractors (GPs) and DHAs' similar role in commissioning services from trusts and other providers. However, this area received less attention and was less rigorously thought through.

The legacy of powers and authority which FHSAs inherited to fulfil any role as purchasers of primary care therefore reflected more closely the agenda of the late 1980s – enhancing the accountability of GPs and the managerial powers of FPCs – than it did the requirements of a true purchasing authority. Only with the outcome of the review of health authorities' function and manpower (Department of Health 1993b) was the nettle finally grasped and it was announced that FHSAs and DHAs would merge to become the integrated purchasers of healthcare, subject to legislation, in 1996.

Information and the purchasing of general medical services

As the purchaser of family health services, the FHSA needs to know:

1 what services are being provided
2 whether services are of acceptable quality
3 whether those services represent a cost effective use of resources
4 and whether services are meeting patients' needs.

These are of course, generic questions for commissioners. Many commentators in the wake of *Working for Patients* commonly perceived them to be pursued best in close conjunction with District Health Authorities in order to achieve good integration between hospital and primary care and good value for money overall. This argument won the day in the functions and manpower review (Department of Health 1993b). The ability of the FHSA to fulfil those tasks reflects:

1 the repertoire of powers granted to it (and the vigour with which these are exercised)
2 the manpower and skills available to it
3 the local managerial and political environment
4 its non-human resources, particularly information technology.

The information routinely available to the FHSA about the volume and type of work general medical practices undertake still reflects the agenda of the late 1980s. FHSAs still remunerate GPs against a centrally negotiated fee scale reflecting the agreed contract (Department of Health 1989c). This payments system constitutes the FHSA's key 'database'. Funds are predominantly allocated from a budget, which is not cash limited, against which GPs claim various payments as of right against the defined *Terms of Service*. It is necessary for the GP only to show that the service has been provided; the FHSA's discretion generally relates only to probity and regularity.

So what can routinely collected data tell the FHSA about the family practitioner services? Almost nothing of value in dentistry since the vast majority of payments to dentists are made by the Dental Estimates Board, and almost nothing about optometrists. While data about drugs dispensed by particular pharmacists is captured by the Prescription Pricing Authority, very little of it is of interest to managers in the family health services field. In general medical practice, however, there is a relatively rich database available, although since it is created for payment purposes its limitations are significant. Notably, the information is most detailed in areas where the *Terms of Service* are specific (and generally, provide for a specific fee to be paid). These are shown in Table 4.1.

For the bulk of services, commonly referred to as 'general medical services' (i.e. the day-to-day consultations between doctor and patient), no data is routinely collected and remitted to the FHSA. The GP is obliged only to notify hours of availability and cover arrangements. The age, sex and address of each patient is held in the database so that capitation payments may be made to the GP and likely demands on general medical services as a consequence of the demographics of a particular list can be deduced. Ethnic origin, however, is not recorded. There is a paucity of data on the bread and butter work of a general practice.

Validation of items of service is difficult and potentially sensitive because of issues of confidentiality. However, examination of the distribution of items of

Table 4.1   Information collected on general medical practice, 1993

Target payments for:

1 childhood immunisations
2 pre-school boosters
3 cervical screening

Whether for each of these areas, each practice reached:

1 No payment target; or
2 The lower target payment; or
3 The upper target payment

in the current quarter and over the whole financial year.

Minor surgery
The number of sessions and individual procedures, conducted in the quarter or over the whole financial year, of the following types:

1 aspirations
2 cautery
3 excisions
4 injections
5 incisions
6 others.

Health promotion clinics
Quarterly and cumulative numbers of sessions held, and the number of individuals attending, analysed by clinical type such as anti-smoking, drug abuse, disease management, diet and exercise and so forth. In the summer of 1993 these clinics were replaced by practice based health promotion programmes associated with the *Health of the Nation* initiative. Practices remit information to the FHSA on their attendance levels and coverage for the health set out in the current guidance documents (NHSME, 1993e).

Night visits
Current quarter and cumulative numbers of visits undertaken, where the visit took place and who visited (i.e. the GP or GP's partner, deputising doctor, etc.).

Maternity medical claims
The number of claims for the quarter and analysis of the type of care delivered such as shared care, GP Unit Confinement, home confinements, post-natal care.

Capitation
An age and sex breakdown of the registered patients. Analysis of how many patients are registered at addresses whose post codes fall into wards with high-, medium- and low-category deprivation.

---

service volume can reveal striking patterns. For example, a GP may appear to spend the majority of his night hours visiting homes in particular streets where all the residents require the urgent attendance from the doctor at some point during the evening! The routine follow-up of strikingly odd distributions of activity such as this will generally be conducted by FHSA staff who may contact patients directly to verify that they have received services, often using their Medical Director to reassure any concerns patients may have about confidentiality. The FHSA may ask practices for information about the rate of return of patients if the amount of activity seems high given the size of cohort in a particular list – for example the number of tetanus jabs in one practice. Such monitoring is politically controversial and has to be undertaken sensitively. Most FHSAs differentiate between the formal follow up of what might appear to be improper claims, usually as a result of an audit exercise or complaint, and the less formal practice visit used to pursue dialogue with practitioners and gather informal intelligence to assess quality of service overall. However, the most important initiative in quality of service in general practice is medical audit, as outlined in the next section.

The FHSA's operational system also provides a limited capacity to review practice performance. The speed and accuracy with which practices return the medical records requested of it, for onward transfer, is a reasonable indicator of a practice's administrative efficiency, particularly if taken with other such routine transactions. Certain other items recorded in the patient database may be of interest to the FHSA. Specifically, the number of patients removed from a GP's list at the GPs request may be monitored to detect adverse selection of patients who represent a particularly heavy workload, such as families requesting a high number of out of hours visits. However the GP is under no formal obligation to give either patient or FHSA an explanation for a removal from his list.

Much of this routine data originates manually at practice level and the accuracy varies. Relatively few practices validate data rigorously although there is a strong incentive for it to be complete because practice income is determined by the claims for payment. The validation of data for capitation purposes is undertaken routinely by FHSAs, particularly since there is no financial incentive for practices to report patients leaving their lists (there is no obligation for a patient to de-register with a GP before moving home and so forth). In an attempt to make capitation payments to GPs correctly, the FHSA may arrange to follow up mail undelivered or unanswered, to obtain information on deaths in the locality, to learn about property demolition and for transient groups such as students to verify their addresses periodically.

Another source of detailed data available to FHSAs since the beginning of the 1990s is the Prescribing Analysis and Costs Tables (PACT). These tables record those prescriptions written by GPs which were subsequently dispensed (a number of prescriptions are never presented to a pharmacist) with an analysis of their costs. FHSAs receive firm drug budgets; while theoretically not cash limited such budgets are subject to increasing scrutiny as efforts are made to contain the explosion of the community drugs bill through the Indicative Prescribing Scheme (Department of Health 1990c). This is a cluster of educational, feedback and budgetary initiatives designed to support and encourage rational prescribing. By examining levels of prescribing of generally cheaper generic products, of particular types of drug, and amounts prescribed, an FHSA can make a relatively sophisticated analysis of this area of clinical activity. This information has only recently been available to FHSAs in computerised format and skills of analysis, particular those of the pharmacist, are relatively newly in place. This is potentially a very powerful means of assessing clinical practice but it also places a substantial workload on information analysis staff.

The FHSA operates a number of services to or on behalf of practices. The accuracy of the patient database is a useful indicator of efficiency of the FHSA's operations. The vast majority of FHSA databases record a higher number of residents than OPCS figures, the difference being known as the 'inflation rate', and this rate can be used with caution as an FHSA performance indicator. The Exeter system provides extremely crude operator performance measurement by counting key strokes, but accurate performance measurement including quality assurance methods such as error logging has to be undertaken manually. Similarly, the timeliness and accuracy with which payments to practitioners are made requires manual recording. These areas of performance are not only of interest to management as indicators of effectiveness and efficiency but they often represent, in practitioners' eyes, the performance and credibility of the FHSA itself.

New FHSA roles

NHS reforms are changing and expanding the roles of FHSAs into such areas as managing the quality of NHS services and attempting to provide primary healthcare on the basis of assessed population needs.

Complaints are commonly used in the hospital and community health services as a way of monitoring quality of service, but this process is problematic in the FHSA. The FHSA has a duty to investigate complaints relating to a family practitioner's fulfilment of the *Terms of Service* and retains local disciplinary powers, pursued in a highly formal quasi-judicial setting and with financial sanctions. Questions of a practitioner's demeanour or professional performance not revealed through a failure to meet specific contractual obligations fall outside the procedures referred to above and the practitioner is under no obligation to cooperate with an FHSA's investigation of them. Nevertheless, the *Patient's Charter* lays a responsibility on FHSAs to investigate all complaints and respond to the complainant (Department of Health 1992). Complaints monitoring can not be used effectively to monitor quality of service of performance until the arrangements for assessing professional performance overall, i.e. dealing with breaches of a practitioner's contract and considering patients' complaints about services generally are clarified.

FHSAs increasingly collect information about consumer satisfaction with primary care services through patient satisfaction surveys or in dialogue with locality groups or Community Health Councils. These methods of obtaining the consumer view can form a helpful backdrop to the development of services although while patients' knowledge of their entitlement to primary care is poorly developed, such an approach must be one of many.

Each FHSA has a Medical Audit Advisory Group (MAAG) which is formally a sub-committee of the FHSA itself (although it may in fact contain no FHSA members). It consists of a locally agreed medical membership, mostly of GPs but with consultants in public health medicine or from the hospital specialities also being involved. In some cases the FHSA's Medical Director or General Manager may be a member or observer at the MAAG. Its function is to lead, stimulate and support medical audit activity at general practice level. It has no formal sanctions should GPs not wish to cooperate. Its resources are granted to it by the FHSA (from its cash limited administration allocation) and FHSAs vary considerably in the level of funding and degree of autonomy granted to MAAGs. The FHSA is entitled to receive the general results of audit, while GP confidentiality is mandated by health circular (HC)(90)15. The FHSA does not therefore receive practice-specific audit results which may be used to gauge the quality of clinical services or the quality of performance of individual GPs or teams. Serious deficiencies revealed to an audit visitor from the MAAG are dealt with in accordance with locally agreed protocols using the professions's existing mechanisms. However the general results of audit, particularly where multi-practice audits are being conducted against locally agreed standards or benchmarks, are useful to the FHSA in its purchasing role. They may point up the need for greater skill availability, for example access to chiropody or dietetics for diabetics receiving their care in general practice, which can be addressed either through the FHSA's own practice staffing resources or through DHA funding. It is, however, the FHSA's responsibility to ensure that its MAAG is successful in obtaining the involvement of all practices in audit and that the audit is conducted to an acceptable standard, despite the confidentiality of specific results and the lack of sanction should GPs decline to participate or do so in only a token fashion.

Under their *Terms of Service*, GPs are required to provide to their FHSA an annual report. While the prescribed content of this report is limited, focusing mainly upon the practice infrastructure and information about the practice's referrals to hospitals, FHSAs invite practices to remit other information about perceived health problems in the locality, initiatives undertaken within the practice, and how the practice intends to develop in the future. It is in the interests of practices to convey this last type of information to the FHSA which is planning its deployment of cash limited resources. Although this kind of information will not be available from all practices and may be subjective and unstructured, it can provide a vital source of intelligence to FHSAs about the extent to which practices are offering a well-balanced response to their population's needs. Only in the case of the small share of limited FHSA resources devoted to reimbursement of practice staffing and premises costs (and its own administration budget) does the FHSA determine how it wishes to use funds. It is in allocating these resources that FHSAs may require further information from GPs in order to support their case for funds.

Questions of the cost effectiveness of individual primary care interventions are not readily investigated using 'gold standard' research or trials. A broader range of approaches is needed. In comparison with hospital services, however, the GP academic and research sectors are small and relatively less well resourced. While the Department of Health has directly funded research on primary care services including a national centre at Manchester from 1994, the proportion of the funds expended in this area has never reflected its central place in the NHS – over 90 per cent of patient contacts with the NHS are estimated to be with the family practitioner services (DHSS 1987).

The requirement on FHSAs to ensure the appropriateness of services to meet the needs of its particular local populace, whether defined by health status, ethnicity or other demographic factors, is not only limited by FHSAs' lack of powers to specify services locally but also by their inability to commission studies which will demonstrate the relative cost effectiveness of different primary care interventions. For example, the respective effectiveness of counsellors or clinical psychologists compared with GPs in dealing with anxiety or other commonly presenting conditions needs to be assessed rigorously if best value for money is to be obtained. A carefully designed programme of research and evaluation such as this is unlikely to be affordable at FHSA level. There are indications that the national research and development strategy being developed by the Department of Health and RHAs (Department of Health 1991) may reflect the need to answer these questions more sensitively than before.

The potential uses of practice-held morbidity data (or similar information held on databases associated with multi-practice medical audits) are being examined by epidemiologists and commissioners with some enthusiasm (Audit Commission 1993). The likelihood of all practices eventually linking electronically to their FHSA/DHA will make the aggregation of data into population profiles possible. Both these developments will enhance the purchasing authority's ability to review services against inferred patient need. However, substantial questions remain to be answered if the potential users of primary care diagnostic and intervention data are to inform purchasing plans, notably the use of a consistent system of coding and classification within general practice (see also Chapter 9). At present the situation is patchy with a number of classifications in use including the Read system (see Chapter 9), Royal College of General Practitioners (RCGP) codes and those associated with particular computer suppliers. Obstacles to the free flow of data of this kind, associated with concerns about confidentiality, will have to be negotiated carefully if GPs are to participate willingly. It will be even more challenging to demonstrate tangible benefits to GPs from their involvement in health needs assessment processes. It is necessary to develop techniques better suited to populations of around 10,000, a typical general practice list size, than traditional epidemiological services. Such developments can only serve to strengthen purchaser–GP relationships and are imperative in the face of the expanding numbers of GP fundholders, if a population based strategic approach to improvements in health status is to be delivered.

Clearly many of the expected changes cannot take place without higher quality information system support. In the next five years the NHS has to move away from these existing conditions:

1 A lack of standards governing many aspects of GP computer systems.
2 About 70 per cent of practices computerised, with wide variations nationally.
3 Only 40 per cent of GPs use a computer in the consulting room; and probably only a minority of these systems are being used for clinical data capture in the patient consultation.
4 A paucity of electronic links between practices, FHSAs, hospitals and other healthcare organisations.
5 Uncertainty about the future of government reimbursement policy.

The information policy goals that all NHS managers and professionals in primary care should be working towards are:

1 Comprehensive, clear standards for the functionality, hardware and data communications capabilities of GP computer systems, agreed by the professions with the Department of Health.
2 Rigorous policing of the standards in connection with an equitable reimbursement policy, which encourages single handed practices to computerise.
3 90 per cent of all practices to be computerised by 1995, the majority of which to be using the computer in face to face contacts with patients.
4 The electronic linking of each GP practice to a network, letting it communicate with any NHS organisation also connected to the network.
5 Collection of morbidity and screening data at practices, using structured protocols and Read Codes, and the sharing of anonymised but personalised data with other NHS bodies.
6 The use of structured messages based on X.400 and EDIFACT communications standards to exchange the majority of information between practices, FHSAs, hospitals and Community Units.

An increasingly urgent task is to review how primary care systems in FHSAs and general practices can best be linked to hospital systems. Chapter

12 sets some of these issues in their health policy context. Meanwhile, the next task is to review the other main information systems to which those in primary care are increasingly linked, the information sytems in NHS trusts.

General practice information systems – progress to date

General practices have a very high level of computerisation relative to other parts of the health service, reflecting a long history and heavy use of computers in the business of general practice. Almost 80 per cent of all general practices make use of computers, with computerised practices having more than two VDUs per partner on average (NHSME 1993b).

Computers in general practice began with a few enthusiasts but as early as 1983 the 'Micros for GPs' scheme encouraged practices to obtain machines and established some of their potential. In 1987 two companies, VAMP and AAH Meditel, introduced 'no cost' computer schemes for general practitioners. GPs were provided with hardware and software at nominal cost in return for morbidity and prescribing data. VAMP began a pilot exercise with 49 practices in 1985 and by the end of the schemes in 1989 each company had about 1000 practices equipped with multiple terminals and prescription printers contributing data on a registered population of five million patients. These schemes gave a considerable hike to GP computerisation and established AAH Meditel and VAMP as leading suppliers – a position they have retained. The schemes were clearly innovative and ambitious but suffered badly from poor data quality as a result of inadequate training and a lack of motivation on the part of the GPs. The wider benefits of aggregating health data from general practice were promoted at the time, but the driving purpose was to produce a profit for the pharmaceutical companies supporting the initiative. The data proved to be deficient for this sole purpose and the 'no cost' scheme was closed in 1991, with the participating practices faced with the choice of buying or losing their computers.

By 1991 GP computing had received another stimulus, its biggest yet. The 1990 GP contract (Department of Health 1989b) paid GPs for reaching specified targets for the proportion of patients immunised or screened for cervical cytology, and for meeting the new requirements to undertake annual health checks on patients aged over 75 and checks every three years on all others. To undertake these activities without a computer system became very laborious in all but the smallest practices. Other developments within the NHS reforms concerned purchasing, medical audit, the greater importance of preventive care and health promotion. These all emphasised the health of populations as well as of individual patients. Much of this responsibility has been placed with GPs through fundholding and the 1993 Health Promotion Package (BMA 1993). GPs are paid to collect lifestyle data and blood pressure readings of their patients – the more patients with a record, the greater the payment. The increasing use of computers in general practice enable theses activities to take place. They require the development of relatively sophisticated information systems.

As a result, 1990 and 1991 saw a tremendous growth in the number of practices with computers, the number of computer suppliers and the use of computers in practices. Levels of computerisation have risen from 10 per cent in 1987, through 63 per cent in 1991 to 79 per cent in 1993. In the 1993 survey, almost 30 per cent of computerised practices already kept full clinical records on their computers with a further 20 per cent actively working towards that goal. Over 90 per cent of practices kept some clinical data, allowing three-quarters of practices to use their computers for audit and one-third for research (NHSME 1993b).

Because such a high level of computerisation has been reached fairly swiftly the market for GP computers has now stabilised considerably as the opportunities for selling new systems become more limited and reimbursement becomes elusive. Whereas there were over 100 suppliers in the boom time just after the introduction of the 1990 contract, there are now about a dozen who would sell a system if asked, plus another 10 or so companies actively selling to GPs. Suppliers can no longer rely upon selling new systems for their income – they must survive on maintenance payments and income from upgrades to existing systems. The long-term profitability of many companies is in serious question.

There has been no standardisation across systems and the choice of system has been left to the individual practice and market forces. It is remarkable that out of this, 70 per cent of practices use one of just six systems. In Scotland, the GPAS system was adopted as the standard, and the majority of computerised Scottish practices have this system. The standard is not compulsory in Scotland, and some have opted for another supplier's system. The Department of Health's 1993 survey and an independent survey of computer usage in Wales confirmed that just about all practices are using their computers for the tasks of registration, repeat prescribing and recalling (Goves et al. 1991; see also below). The Welsh survey highlighted the extent to which GPs fail to make use of their systems to anything like their potential, but also their firm intentions to make more use of them in the future.

So there is a plethora of different systems in use with whole variety of coding systems and operating platforms. The capabilities of the different systems reflect their history and original purpose. The Meditel and VAMP systems arose out of the prescribing and morbidity data collection schemes; many of the subsequent systems have concentrated upon meeting the requirements of the 1990 contract. The newest systems attempt a clinical record together with comprehensive management functions.

Functions of general practice information systems

All GP computer systems for managing primary healthcare are based upon a database built from the individual patient record. The major systems allow the recording and retrieval of registration, prescribing, diagnoses, symptoms, physiological measurements, occupation and referral data, together with administrative data relating to claims for payment and recalling patients for screening and monitoring. The three 'Rs' of GP systems are registration, repeat prescribing, and recalling. Registration data is required to even have a patient on the system, and is the basis of all other uses of the computer. Repeat prescribing and recalling by computer allows the potential for greater control and efficiency. Equally, there is the increased potential for errors and omissions to go unnoticed, as with any partially automated operation. The three 'Rs' can be achieved by a single screen and printer in the practice office. The proliferation of VDUs on doctors' desks in the consulting room, together with the urge to maintain a full clinical record confirms that the extent of computerisation is still increasing rapidly and that more uses are being found for them in practice.

A GP using a computer for recording a consultation is doing two things. First, she is making a record that she, or another member of the primary care team, will want to see again at some time in the future about that patient. This first record need be no different from the written record in the Lloyd George envelope. But secondly, the GP is making entries into a patient database which may be searched and information retrieved from it. The two functions are very different, but in keeping with the IM&T strategy principle of deriving information from operational systems (see Chapter 2), the aim must be to combine them as much as possible. An uncoded free text entry on the computer is perfectly adequate for the first use, but of very limited use for analysis. Equally a bald Read code (see Chapter 9) without any text does not tell you anything about that individual patient, but is all that is required for analysis. By making fully coded entries, supplemented with free text comments of no consequence to the database, but of real value in the care of an individual patient, both requirements are met. These principles are universal, but are particularly pertinent to the recording of clinical consultations, with the pressures of time and the fluid mix of hard physiological measurement, clinical diagnosis and anecdotal reminders.

The computerised clinical record brings a number of benefits even in the consultation, quite apart from the contribution it makes to the database. The computer allows the clinician clearer and more flexible access to the record. There are many old jokes about the legibility of doctors' handwriting, based soundly upon truth. Many GPs have difficulty discerning their own partners' writing. Combine this with drastically abbreviated medical jargon and the result is a written record which is only meaningful to the original author. The computerised record is first of all readable, with many abbreviations expanded to make them accessible to a wider audience. The clinician can make rapid selective retrieval of notes of a particular type (such as medication, laboratory results and operations), and also view only those entries relevant to one particular problem. In this way, more careful consideration can be made of the patient's clinical history resulting in improved diagnosis and planning of therapies and care.

Many GPs have the screen in a position that allows the patient to see it too, giving the patient the opportunity to question the content of the record and obtain a more satisfactory explanation from the clinician. This alters the power relationships in the consultation and allows the patient to feel more involved and responsible for the care or therapy recommended. The record is also more likely to be accurate. Prescriptions printed on computer are also legible – by patients, pharmacists and carers.

GP computer systems increasingly offer a modicum of decision support. They do not pretend to be 'expert systems' making the clinician redundant, but prompt the clinician for data, offer reminders and check for impossible entries, such as a diastolic blood pressure of 300 mm/hg. Similarly, data collection protocols can be defined that interact with data already in the record and with entries as they are made. For example, a prompt for the smoking history of a patient with asthma may be presented only if one does not already exist in the record for the last 12 months. This increases the quality of the data in the database, but also helps the clinician at the time to collect an appropriate history and conduct an appropriate examination, without fear of unnecessary repetition or unintentional omission. The drug databases incorporate warnings that present themselves automatically when patients are about to be prescribed a drug that interacts unfavourably with their existing medication. Also, sensitivities to a particular medication can be entered in such a way that any attempt to issue an item with a congruent component causes an alert to be displayed. These attributes of the system are transparent to the user. They only manifest themselves when an oversight is made. In normal use, the clinician is not constantly bombarded with warnings, prompts and alerts.

The benefits of using the computer rather than written notes in the consultation are themselves valuable, but also the necessary bait to capture the data to provide a comprehensive, rich database from which even greater value can be obtained. Ideally, all consultations will be recorded on the computer, but great steps can be taken by recording a data from patients fulfilling a limited set of criteria. For example, a practice may decide to record all consultations with patients suffering from the chronic diseases of asthma, diabetes and hypertension only, as a step towards full electronic clinical records. The GP system eases the task of operating a recall system for those patients with chronic diseases, so that it becomes easier to set up clinics for a wider range of conditions, and easier to identify defaulters. Similarly, the easy identification of at risk groups allows them to be targeted for specific care, screening, or prevention therapies.

A major value of GP computer systems beyond the three 'Rs' is easing the task of medical audit. The audit cycle starts with setting objectives or standards of care, followed by data collection, analysis and review to assess behaviour by those standards. The cycle is completed with a decision to implement change in order to come closer to the standard. Often the bulk of audit effort is concentrated on collecting and analysing data, to the extent that audit is mistakenly viewed as these activities alone. The routine collection of data onto a computer system provides the possibility of what Paul Bradley calls 'painless audit' (Bradley 1993). Computer systems can be engineered to collect, analyse and present data regularly and almost automatically, allowing clinicians to concentrate upon the more productive tasks of setting objectives and implementing change. This ease of operation drives the audit cycle around and around, allowing a pace of change capable of keeping up with patient, clinician and government demand (Mackintosh and Bradley 1993). Audit becomes integral to the management of the practice, not an extra chore or sideline issue.

As the scope of data on the system increases – from repeat prescribing to acute prescribing, chronic diseases, screening, background lifestyle data, laboratory and imaging results and eventually routine morbidity, so the scope of the potential audits also increases. Audit can be conducted across a wide variety of clinical conditions, but also within any one condition, the audit can address the clinical, managerial and even financial aspects of the problem. A comprehensive database can provide multiple perspectives on processes and activities which can give clear indicators of health outcome, although true outcome measures will always remain elusive, especially in primary care. The challenge is no longer the collection of data, but the incorporation of the derived information into the healthcare process.

Mention has already been made of GPs' increased responsibilities for the health of their practice population, not just the individuals in that population. This responsibility is exercised most vigorously in fundholding practices and those involved in practice-based commissioning. These practices have to make choices about the health needs of their practice populations, a duty that can only be carried out adequately with an effective computerised information system. Health status and health needs data at district and electoral ward level are insufficiently precise and sensitive for decisions at this scale. The task of health needs assessment often includes attempts at guessing the health status of a population from hospital, mortality, social and consumer statistics. Much of the data on GP computer systems could provide very much more precise, accurate and relevant information from which to build a needs assessment.

Already some practices could provide a continuous demographic and morbidity profile of the practice population, backed up by a high level of recording of smoking, alcohol consumption, exercise activity, family history and Body Mass Index. The incidence and prevalence of health problems presented to the practice clinicians can be available regularly. Prescribing, drug addiction, symptoms, a smattering of social status data, and the number of attendances to the practice for each condition contribute further to what could already be a very full assessment of the health needs of the practice population. This information can be available for all ages and all health problems – not just for a selected few. The number of attendances for a particular problem suggests its effect on the patient and so is a crude but effective measure of patient demand. The 'lifestyle' data gives a measure of clinical need, as yet unexpressed as patient demand. The need for services from the secondary sector is very crudely measured with referral rates for each speciality.

For a full health needs assessment, information must be obtained on the range of care services available and the effectiveness of that care. Significant steps can be made towards this by somehow extending the scope of the data on the GP system to include data from patient consultations taking place outside the practice. GPs receive reports about their patients from hospitals, almost invariably in the form of a discharge letter. To make use of this properly it must be interpreted, coded and keyed into the GP system. Many practices do so, in order to monitor what hospital treatments their patients receive. A full picture of care can only be obtained if all patient encounters with other carers – GPs, practice clinicians, paramedics, hospital clinicians, community staff and social services – are also recorded. It would then be possible, for example, to select any condition and see what therapy the practice gave, how many patients were referred to hospital, what they had done to them there and, following discharge, what care they had from community and social services. Finally, and most importantly, one could see whether they presented to the GP again with the same condition. Information of this richness allows proper planning and allocation of care between the general practice, community, secondary and even social services.

Unfortunately, many of the data to support this kind of information do not enter the practice in any form and so special arrangements have to be made to capture them. While the Community Information System for Purchasers (CISP) have explored links between community health services and general practice, this has usually consisted of feeding back selective paper-based information from the community system. This is a long way from integrating information systems. The only way that the analyses outlined above can be carried out is if GP and community patient data coexist on one system – preferably the GP one. Building information links with social services is yet more difficult. Only a minority of referrals to social services originate in general practice and so stand a chance of being recorded there. Many social services departments do not record clients' registered GP on their systems. Without these data it is difficult even to make a start on the above analyses, as it is impossible to identify which patients a practice needs data about.

Whatever the scope of data capture in individual general practices, the information derived from GP systems is certainly of benefit to individual practices wishing to audit their provision of General Medical Services. It can also assist them in purchasing or commissioning health services from elsewhere. The potential for auditing, planning, purchasing and managing health services on a larger scale using these data is only beginning to be realised.

Implementing and developing general practice information systems

The spread of GP information systems described above seems to have encouraged enthusiasm and innovation, making the development and acceptance of GP computing a success story. The major problem now perceived by the Department of Health is that incompatible systems inhibit the sharing of information. In order to ensure the wise investment of public money in GP computing and coherent future development, the NHSME has defined a set of minimum national requirements to be met by all GP computer systems (NHSME-IMG 1993a), formally implemented from 1 April 1994. There is no doubt that further functionality and standardisation will be defined into these requirements in the future.

A multi-user GP computing system costs on average £15000 to purchase and £2500 a year to maintain. This is equivalent to a purchase cost of around £3 per registered patient plus £1 per patient annual maintenance and upgrade costs. Unit costs are greater for small practices, and very much greater for fundholding practices which require extra software and higher specification hardware. Most practices now own their computer whereas renting was more common a couple of years ago, particularly under the 'no cost' schemes.

A proportion of purchase, maintenance and initial staff costs have been eligible for reimbursement from the FHSA since 1989. This scheme initially set a maximum sum that could be reimbursed, depending on the size of practice. This maximum has now been removed but the amount and level of reimbursement are now at FHSA discretion. The stated level of reimbursement is 50 per cent, or 75 per cent for equipment related to fundholding. However, computer reimbursement monies in the FHSAs are cash limited. The actual reimbursement levels vary wildly between FHSAs and between practices governed by the same FHSA. Priority for reimbursement is given to fundholding practices, those buying a system for the first time, and for equipment for the GP-FHSA links project. Computer costs will only be reimbursed for systems that meet the *Requirements for Accreditation*, which FHSAs are not permitted to 'interpret' locally. The requirements are that a GP computer system:

1 uses Read codes (see Chapter 9)
2 includes a drug database maintained by the supplier

3 can computerise practice formularies
4 has a full audit trail
5 supports GP–FHSA links.

These features arise from the need for GP systems to comply with the *NHS Information Management and Technology (IM&T) Strategy* (NHSME-IMG 1992; see Chapters 2 and 12), particularly with regard to standardised coding and communications. They also reflect the Department of Health's desire to see computerised clinical records become acceptable for medico-legal purposes, and for GP computer systems to assist in cost-effective prescribing. They will undoubtedly lead to a further decline in the number of suppliers. It is quite possible that no more than half a dozen different systems will be in active use within a few years.

Information systems for general practice fundholding

A fundholding practice requires a relatively sophisticated clinical information system for monitoring and planning its provision and purchase of care. Only once this system is delivering high quality information can the practice make sensible decisions about where to allocate its fund. Operational monitoring of the fund must by law take place on a computer using software written to the Department of Health's specification. The original specification for the fundholding software was produced by a firm of accountants in the autumn of 1990 and suppliers had to produce working software for the 300 or so first wave fundholding practices by 1 April 1991. GP computer suppliers have had to submit their software for conformance testing against the Department of Health specification. One GP computer supplier still has to devote a third of its development resources to fundholding, much of it simply keeping up with the changing specification. This does not leave much for embellishments and innovation.

The fundholding software was written to ensure accountability in the use of public funds, not to ease the management of those funds in general practice. The software collects the necessary data to provide the statutory monthly financial statements to the FHSA. It is very much an accountancy tool and some experience of financial statements is required to gain much information from the outputs. Version 2 of the software, required by the Department of Health from 1 April 1993, allows for the inclusion of contracts for community services and for fuller reporting.

The software serves its purpose but needs large volumes of data to service it, necessitating substantial clerical resources. Yet the software, even in its later versions, still cannot report on much of the most valuable data. For example, the fundholding software specification does not of itself stipulate reports on the number of initial referrals from the practice to each speciality at each provider unit. This is a basic set of information used for fixing the size of the fund in the first place and for subsequent monitoring of the use of the fund. Neither does the software identify patients waiting for inpatient treatments, even though the data are in there somewhere.

Different GP computer suppliers have provided their own add-ons to the basic specification, often allowing more flexible reporting. However, this has not developed sufficiently to allow the fundholding software to be a comprehensive fund management tool. No supplier offers a fundholding system fully integrated with their clinical system. They may share the same hardware, share the same registration database and even make some entries in the clinical record, but they are not integrated. Operations performed in hospital and entered in the fundholding software for charging purposes will not show up in a search on the clinical system. To start with, the fundholding software works on OPCS codes whereas most of the clinical systems work on Read codes (see Chapter 9). A fully integrated system should allow a search on a defined group of patients (for example diabetics or infants) to show what demands they made on the practice fund, and from which providers. Only when the fundholding software can do this will it be possible to match resources to need effectively.

The development of information systems for general practice

Two forces are likely to drive the technical development of GP computer systems. One is the annual review of the Requirements for Accreditation. The other is market competition among suppliers. Accreditation of GP computer systems has brought in no small element of standardisation. This makes it easier for GPs to change their software without losing their data. As a result it is increasingly necessary for suppliers to improve their product in order to stay in business. Sometimes the two forces for development are not exerted in the same direction. For example it is a Department of Health requirement that systems display the prices of drugs that are prescribed but one computer supplier found that two-thirds of its users positively did not want this information displayed on screen.

Because GPs have been almost a captive market in the past the software supplied to them has not been very user-friendly. It could not compete with the pretty products in the worlds of commerce or finance. While hardware costs may make full graphical user interfaces unlikely for a time, all suppliers are seeking ways to improve this area. The value of the computer in the consultation room can be increased through easier access and clearer presentation of selected aspects of the patient record, such as changes in physiological measurements over time. There is scope for greater use of decision support, building in clinical protocols based on national or practice guidelines. The concept of a clinical workstation is probably of more value to a GP than to doctors in other environments and research by the Manchester Medical Information Group is demonstrating its practicability. Suppliers are also actively considering further purely technical developments such as remote access to practice while the doctor is on visits, and electronic 'pen and pad' systems.

The loudest cry from GPs is for links between their information systems and others, in laboratories, hospitals, FHSAs and elsewhere. These developments are the most difficult as they require the same standards at the practice, at the remote site and for the link in between. Many pilot projects are exploring the placing of laboratory test results directly into GP computer systems and it is likely that this will become commonplace. Similarly hospital discharge summaries can be entered electronically. The link can go the other way too, allowing GPs to book patients appointments in hospitals.

These developments will ease the use of computers and produce operational efficiencies. However, the most revolutionary developments will probably come from the new information that properly managed GP information systems can make available, particularly when that information is aggregated across practices. When VAMP and AAH Meditel abandoned their practice data collection schemes in 1991 and 1993 a number of other organisations stepped in to take over collection from a smaller number of practices. The majority of these are pharmaceutical companies who still value the data but require it on a reduced scale. The collapse of the AAH Meditel scheme also saw the launch of the Doctors' Independent Network (DIN). This is an organisation of doctors who wish to see these data used for audit and resource management at practice, locality, district and larger scales, and yet be certain that doctors maintain ownership of the data for the sake of confidentiality and the maintenance of patient trust. DIN is spearheading developments in electronic communications and data aggregation from practices across the country in advance of standardisation that will arise from the accreditation requirements. Even with only just over a hundred practices connected to the network, DIN is developing uses for the information for audit, education, research, epidemiology and pharmaco-epidemiology. Innovations in these areas will exploit the true value of GP computer systems – the diligent recording of individual patient consultations that can enable effective healthcare provision for much larger populations.

Chapter 5

TRUST INFORMATION SYSTEMS

Norman Ambage

Introduction

In any organisation, whether a business, a charitable institution or an NHS hospital, good information is crucial to decision making and effective management. Since the aggregation of the various managerial decisions taken over time will determine hospital cost-effectiveness the latter largely depends on the quality of information available to managers. While managerial decisions can be made (and sometimes are) on the basis of little or no information, it is unlikely that *good* decisions can be made without accurate, timely and relevant information.

Sentiments similar to those above have been expressed by various bodies within (and without) the NHS over the past few years. They were seen as crucial in the drive to inject a more 'business-like' approach into the running of the NHS. These concepts were turned into reality first by the Griffiths proposals (DHSS 1983) and the fumbling Management Budgeting experiment, and then following the launch of the Resource Management Initiative (RMI) in 1986 and the implementation of *Working for Patients* in 1989, which included such revolutionary ideas as the internal market, the purchaser–provider split, and GP fundholding. In this maelstrom of pressurised development, enormous changes have occurred in the information required to manage a hospital, in the personnel demanding the information, and in systems designed to deliver that information.

The central tenets of information have, of course, remained unchanged since pre-Körner days – information must be credible, timely, complete and accurate. For it to be more managerially useful, however, it must also be easily retrievable, multi-disciplinary (in both clinical and non-clinical terms), relevant, and malleable. Computerisation, often on a vast scale, is a necessity. This much was recognised in the RMI. The RMI, designed to 'improve the quality and quantity of patient care through the better use of resources' (Baird 1992) had two central pillars: directly involving doctors, nurses and other clinicians in the management of the hospital by creating the necessary managerial environment (often using the directorate model); and creating an information system that was accessible and credible to all. At the heart of this information vision lay the Case Mix Management System (CMMS). Six sites were chosen to pilot the ideas contained in the concept of the RMI (Arrowe Park Hospital, the Freeman Hospital, Guy's Hospital, Huddersfield Royal Infirmary, Pilgrim Hospital Boston, and the Royal Hampshire County Hospital). Aside from considerable cultural convulsions, monies were lavished on information systems with varying degrees of success. In 1989, it was announced that Resource Management had moved from the experimental stage to one that was to be rolled out across the whole of the NHS. In 1991 researchers at Brunel University concluded that it was not possible to provide a clear assessment of the efficacy of the RMI and that it was equally impossible to isolate any measurable improvements in patient care (Robinson 1991). Many managers disagreed with the general tone of the Brunel findings, arguing that the much greater involvement of medical staff in the management of resources and in planning services was (and is) in itself a major step forward in hospital management.

In 1994, Resource Management is continuing to be implemented within acute units though experience has shown that it is often difficult fully to realise the theoretical potential of CMMS (see below). The launch of *Working for Patients* (Department of Health 1989a) further increased the demand for management information with the establishment of the internal market and the purchaser–provider split (in part also providing the motivation for the accelerated roll out of the RMI). Concise and timely patient-based data were required for billing purposes (especially where cost and volume or cost per case contracts were in place, and particularly in the case of ECRs). It did not take providers of healthcare long to realise that money did not, after all, follow the patient, but was much more likely to follow the patient's data. In short, managers soon learnt that no data meant no money.

As contracting has developed within the NHS, other information gaps have appeared: marketing intelligence; contract monitoring; activity modelling; and costing and pricing data. Further initiatives have been added to the original RMI and these too have demanded the presence of good information: medical and clinical audit, the *Patient's Charter*, and Total Quality Management (TQM). In response to these further demands, greater reliance has been placed on ever-larger and more sophisticated computer systems, in particular on Hospital Information Support Systems (HISS). Whereas the RMI helped create an environment for significant developments within the information field, the internal market has both fully exploited that new environment and provided a cloche for further rapid development. As the RMI roll out from its six pilot sites roughly coincided with the start of the NHS internal market, the two developments are often erroneously seen as one and the same (Baird 1993). But this is to run ahead of ourselves a little. For the moment it is enough to note the typical range and types of information needed to manage hospital cost effectiveness, quality and activity.

Customers for information

While there are as many different business needs within the NHS as there are hospitals, there is enough commonality to sustain useful comments on general information requirements. Within most provider units there are four major 'customers' for information: central government and its representatives including the Department of Health, regions and NHSME outposts (until 1986) purchasers, including consortia, DHAs, FHSAs and GP fundholders; internal customers, especially clinical directorates and contracting departments; and various miscellaneous customers, including those involved in quality initiatives, audit and care in the community.

From the above list, it is fairly clear that there are some 'old' customers (like the Department of Health), albeit wearing slightly different hats, and a large number of new customers – GP fundholders, clinical directorates, contracting departments. Each has distinctly different needs. For example, purchasers require information on only 'their' particular patients (whether residence or GP practice based) and demand patient-based data sets (whether electronic or manual) to support billing and activity monitoring. The Department of Health and regions continue to require Körner-type data, but have added various 'fast track' data collection activities, especially concerning waiting-list information. They also demand breakdowns by residence for many of the standard returns. The growth in 'businesses' within each hospital (directorates), with their attendant business managers, has created a whole new pool of information-hungry staff and their needs are bounded only by the imagination of the enquirer. But perhaps the most voracious user of data and information in any healthy provider unit is the contracting department.

So the role of Unit Information Teams has also had to be revolutionised in response to RMI and the introduction of internal markets. Previously the *raison d'etre* of information teams was to 'feed the beast' at the Department of Health. Now their duties encompass support to in-house managers – indeed, this aspect of information work ought to be the major business of any unit information team. It is as well to appreciate that Department of Health duties carry on (indeed have grown), but these should be carried out 'in the background', as mere routine. In many cases this change in workload emphasis has also meant a change in the character of information personnel – away from traditional clerks and the mere transferral of manually collected data to the appropriate central return, to highly computer literate information professionals who see analysis and advice as the major pillars of their work. The success or failure of unit information staff can be judged by how far they have travelled along the road of transition and how responsive they are to the demands of in-house managers.

Data, information needs and information systems

One problem facing most trust information teams is to satisfy disparate information needs from inflexible (and often parlous) systems originally designed to cater only for the requirements of the centre. For trusts which were not original RMI sites much effort (often ingenious) is expended in trying to transform systems into something which they were never designed to be – the joining of daily battle with ageing and/or manual systems is common.

Here one must recall the distinction between 'data' and 'information' (see Chapter 1). Much of what is said about improving NHS 'information' systems is really about improving data collection systems (though some data are more informative than others). Data are first collected (whether manually or electronically), then selected, analysed, manipulated and presented to become the first form of information proper. The second, more important stage in generating information is assessment. This cannot be done by machine but only in the mind of the user. Producing information is essentially a human process.

Of data there are in hospitals four basic kinds: activity, financial, manpower and clinical. Each is important in its own right, and when brought together form a powerful managerial tool. Historically, different departments have dealt with these four different kinds of data. Thus the local trust information team will probably deal only with activity data (how many inpatients and day cases were admitted, how many patients passed through the A&E department, etc.). Financial data come under the jurisdiction of the finance department, manpower data under personnel, and clinical data are largely held in case notes (with a small amount on the Patient Administration System (PAS) and departmental systems). So for most information teams their title is something of a misnomer – mostly they deal only in activity information.

Sources of data (as opposed to information) exist in abundance at hospital level. Unfortunately, many of these sources are rarely audited and often do not conform to any national standard. While many manual (and a few computerised) data sources bear rich, managerially relevant seams of information, there must always be doubt when consulting any local, unmanaged data source. Conversely, most computerised data collection systems, if run along correct lines, will hold masses of standard items, accessible by standard reports, but may be rather less managerially useful. Bearing these caveats in mind, data sources range from manual systems (nursing diaries, card indexes of one sort or another, handwritten A&E (accident and emergency department) logs, theatre books, etc.) through microcomputers at local level, to mini- and mainframe computers at trust, District and Regional level. More specialised sources of data exist at hospital department level: for radiology, pathology, therapies, theatres, etc. Important human sources of data include the trust information team, the finance department, the department of human resources (personnel), the local public health department, the DHA information team and other hospital business managers. While they last, Regional Health Authorities also have information teams. Regional and national publications can be of great value: *OPCS Monitor* (detailing such things as live births, notifications of infectious diseases, and newly diagnosed communicable diseases, by county), *Vital Statistics* (showing births by age group, mortality statistics, and infant mortality rates, by District Health Authority and electoral ward), *Public Health Data Sets* and *Health Service Indicators* are just a few.

Leaving aside the non-standardised and heavily manual data collection points outlined above, the following are the major sources of standard data.

Patient administration system (PAS)

One of the richest seams of data, PAS holds patient-based records dealing with a wide range of demographic data, hospital activity data (waiting list, outpatient and inpatient or day case information), an array of other useful indicators such as method and source of admission, destination on discharge and method of discharge and contractual data, together with a small amount of clinical information usually in the form of diagnostic and procedure (operation) codes. Unfortunately, these systems are often fairly inflexible and only standard reports emanate directly from them. The newer PASs with more recently available interrogation tools can provide a more flexible query base. More often than not, though, reports direct from PAS are used merely to feed Department of Health standard returns or are downloaded to standard software packages to produce a more sensitive and relevant routine monitoring reports for in-house or departmental consumption. Managerially useful reports can be forthcoming from these systems depending upon how old they are or how ingenious the local IT or information team has been.

PASs are the commonest operation systems in acute hospitals and have been in place for some time. They usually consist of a suite of integrated modules. A patient registration module maintains the person (e.g. names, date of birth, sex) and administrative details (e.g. general practice, home address) of patients treated at the hospital. These details are held in a master patient index (MPI). This should obviously play a key role in virtually all hospital activity, allowing information about the individual patient to be captured or updated once on initial contact with the hospital and then made available to other systems supporting the delivery of specific items or packages of care. MPI is essentially the hospital's consumer list.

A PAS inpatient management module is designed to support the delivery of care to patients admitted as day cases or for overnight stays. It should assist the effective use of hospital resources, especially beds and support services, by recording which patient is in which ward under the care of which clinician. This module holds information on whether the patient has been admitted from the waiting list and details of when, where and how he or she has been discharged. It provides key management information on the hospital's workload. In most PASs the outpatient module is essentially an appointment system for scheduling clinics. It records planned appointments for individual patients and indicates whether the patient attended. Not all hospital clinics have implemented such booking systems yet.

Department systems

Departmental systems are often not patient-based and can be intensely manual. They again hold basic patient demographic data (name, address, age, sex, etc.) and data pertinent to the relevant department. For a comprehensive list of what data such a system collects, what standard reports it produces and for advice on the efficacy of any *ad hoc* report-writing tools one should approach either the trust information manager or the system manager for the department. Nevertheless, the more common departmental systems are recognisably similar in different hospitals.

Radiology systems generally automate the referral, booking and scheduling of patient appointments; record radiological investigation results; schedule equipment and facilities use (hence maintenance, etc.); control stocks of consumables; and help maintain patient records. Typically data will include basic patient demographics (again), GP details, status of examination (routine, urgent), sources of examination requests (A&E, outpatients, other hospital, etc), consultant details, where in the hospital the examination was carried out (A&E department, ultrasound, etc.), examination details (right lateral chest, radius and ulna, sinuses and antra, etc.), and Körner codes. Pathology systems automate the ordering and scheduling of laboratory tests (and record requests for them); report test results (often automatically); and monitor laboratory equipment performance and stocks of laboratory supplies. Pharmacy systems normally process drug orders and prescriptions (usually issues to wards rather than to individual patients), dispensing and stock control. Theatre management systems normally schedule operations, theatre sessions and the resources required; control theatre supply stocks; and schedule equipment maintenance. Data collected will typically include patient types (daycase, inpatient, etc.); anaesthetic and operative procedures (in OPCS4 or Read codes – see Chapter 9); when operations began and ended, and the staff involved; how much time each patient spent in the recovery suite; and outcomes (including nosocomial infections). Nursing systems usually automate the scheduling of nursing staff (rotas, etc.), record staff absences, and automate the planning of nurse training.

Financial systems

Financial systems tend to hold a vast array of data relating to the general ledger, stores transactions, budgets, accounts payable, billing and debtors. Three areas are of major interest for clinical directors, business or general managers. 'Accounts payable' records such things as the names of vendors, payment details, invoice and order number. The general ledger holds details of transactions and calculates current and cumulative budget positions from whole-trust level through directorates down to the smallest department. Billing and debtors, and stores transactions systems (holding details on commodities ordered, their quantity, value, transfer point, financial code, etc.), are part of the central financial system in some trusts but not others. Financial systems invariably have an extensive suite of standard reports and tools to modify them. Standard reports should split budgets into monies for salaries and wages by staff grade, for consumables, travel, etc. More modern systems have extremely flexible and user-friendly *ad hoc* report writers. There appears no reason why network access to these tools cannot be made available to managerial staff.

Manpower and personnel systems

Manpower and personnel systems hold employee-based data with rich demographic data including qualifications, payroll data and special attributes. Data are often collected by downloading from the personal system and can show such things as overtime reports and nominal staff rolls. Also included will be individuals' service history, pay allowances, disciplinary details, source of recruitment, destination on leaving and reasons for leaving. Post details include source of funding, payscale, site and cost centre. Links to financial systems provide budgetary analyses of manpower use. Most data are coded using national and local codes and the more modern systems have reasonably sensitive analysis tools to provide manpower information for managers.

Clinical information systems

Little clinical information exists in the systems so far described. There may be small amounts in each departmental system (diagnoses and operative procedures in PAS, radiological examinations in X-Ray systems, blood tests in pathology, etc.) but by itself each system is clinically poor in terms of the whole patient. Some hospitals have specific clinical information systems that sit astride other systems, or there may be a CMMS. Otherwise the most likely source of clinically rich data is the case note (see Chapter 8). Of course, these case notes are often cumbersome, lost, in the boot of the doctor's car, in transit or indecipherable. All are intensely manual. For any kind of detailed clinical audit trawling through innumerable case notes by hand is probably the only course of action available.

For the future much emphasis is being placed on creating electronic medical records (see Chapter 9). Computerised medical histories could contain textual, visual and aural information, could be stored on optical disc and retrieved from a 'juke-box' via a computer terminal. Such systems are being developed in the UK and USA.

Generally, there are problems associated with all the above 'first port of call' information systems and the situation regarding case note data tends to highlight them. These widespread difficulties involve information retrieval and information linking. NHS 'information' systems find it reasonably easy to collect data but not so easy to retrieve information flexibly or to link to other systems. In more modern environments such as mature hospital information support system sites (HISS) or sites with a reasonably well established and well run CMMS flexible access to multi-disciplinary data might well be more easily achieved than on the more traditional site.

Case mix management system (CMMS)

Managers in trusts with a mature CMMS benefit greatly from improved access to multi-disciplinary data. A CMMS can be linked to a giant mixing pot of sub-sets of data from all the above systems. The data are patient-based so it is possible to obtain a whole-patient picture ranging in theory from basic demographics through operative procedures performed, X-Rays taken and drugs prescribed, to physiotherapy carried out, follow-up outpatient care and even care in the community (if the necessary feeder systems and interfaces exist). Most importantly, these individual patient profiles of longitudinal data can be aggregated to present high-level views of hospital businesses while retaining the ability to 'drill-down' to various sub-levels. Manpower and financial data can be linked with rich and extensive clinical information from a single database, using technology requiring only limited computing or programming skills.

Many CMMSs also have an executive information system (EIS) attached. EISs accept large volumes of data from host machines and, after a substantial amount of background work by either the IT department or the information team, offer extremely user-friendly front ends to complicated computer systems. Often these EISs exist primarily as a graphic interface, but retain the ability to produce statistical reports and 'drill down' to the next level of data detail. EISs need not exist only as part of a CMMS but can be adapted to use with most computer systems.

Sites with a mature, fully functioning CMMS are few. Most trusts with a CMMS can boast a case mix system with PAS data and perhaps one or two additional feeders (usually theatres and radiology with some limited financial data). Some CMMS sites have only just combined PAS data with their case mix data. It would be wise to check with the local IT or information manager as to the progress made with any CMMS that might be available. If a CMMS is available – use it!

Hospital information support systems (HISS)

Shortly after the Resource Management Initiative began the HISS programme was initiated. Its aims were to test the 'feasibility of specifying, procuring and implementing systems which would cover every operational and information need of acute general hospitals . . . bringing together the separate operational systems . . . into a single integrated system'. A handful of sites were used to 'pilot' the HISS idea – Greenwich District, Darlington Memorial and the City (Nottingham) hospitals. HISS seeks to supply computerised information support facilities for most hospital functions: medical records, PAS, case mix, order entry, results reporting, radiology, pathology, nurse rostering, theatres, A&E, contracting, billing and care planning, using a common Master Patient Index as its focal point. Such integrated systems require data to be entered only once and provide information from a common data source to all levels of the organisation – general managers, clinicians, operational and support staff, etc. The database is updated by transferring information from the hospital's operational systems. Its comprehensiveness therefore depends on which systems 'feed' it. HISSs are designed to allow standard costs to be recorded for particular tests or items of care, building up a picture of the resources used to treat individuals or groups of patients. They also allow clinicians to record what profiles of treatment they would expect certain types of patient to receive, and to compare these with what actually happens to patients. Thus the quality of decision making, together with the quality of service provided, should improve.

The original HISS sites sought the wholesale replacement of their existing systems – the so-called 'big bang' approach. However, the NHS Information Management Group now promulgates an 'incremental' route to HISS, making as much use as possible of existing systems. The problem here is that many extant systems are old and overburdened – to try to teach them new tricks is often extremely difficult. For many IT and information managers seeking a way forward into HISS, upgrading their ancient Patient Administration Systems is the priority. Nevertheless, the IM&T strategy (see Chapter

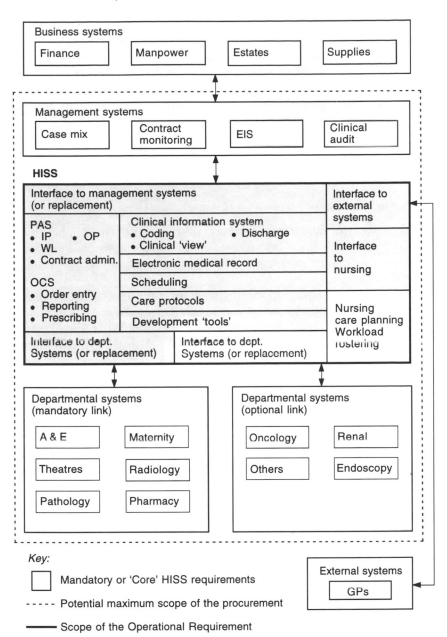

Figure 5.1 Overview of a total hospital information system: an example
Source: Kwo, D. and Cruickshank, J., HISS: practical progress at the leading edge, in Richards (ed.) (1994) p. 362

2) set a target of the year 2000 for all large acute hospitals to have an integrated system. To help this, 'framework' agreements have been reached with computer companies. These agreements allow companies to supply similar products to listed customers without the buyers having to embark upon the protracted EU procurement process (see Chapter 11). At present 'framework' contracts apply only to hospitals of less than 400 beds. In 1992 Kidderminster became the first HISS 'framework' site.

Not many trusts have a mature, fully functioning HISS – though many have started on the programme. Advice should be sought from the IT or information manager as to the current status of any HISS.

Contract management system

With the advent of the internal market, contracting systems are becoming increasingly important to NHS managers. As contracting within the NHS is evolving, so are contract management systems. At present there is no single definitive system.

There are three main parts to such a system. Its contract allocation function generally forms part of PAS and allocates each patient activity to a particular contract. For example, inpatient and day case allocation will take place after clinical coding has been completed. Among other things, the PAS contracting algorithms will take account of the patient's postcode, the intended management, the source and method of admission, the GP and the operative procedure. A combination of such factors automatically produces a contract identification number and allocates the patient activity to a particular contract. A manual override is also often built into these systems to sort out definitional problems or to reflect any locally made agreements.

Secondly, the system should produce contract minimum data sets (CMDS) for billing the relevant purchaser, together with any PAS-generated aggregate activity reports. CMDS contain the minimum amount of data required to support the billing and monitoring process. They are:

1 patient specific data (name, address, post code, GP, etc.)
2 referral details (for outpatients), or
3 spell details (for inpatients and day cases) – admission date, management intention, discharge date, etc., and
4 attendance details (for outpatients), or episode details (for inpatients) – consultant name, speciality, episode start and end dates, clinical codes.

These data can be sent directly to a billing and debtors system to generate bills for sending electronically or on paper to the purchaser.

Thirdly, some (not all) CMMS have in-built contract monitoring systems. These become important when dealing with GP fundholders, each of whom normally has his or her own contract with the trust. Trusts without CMMS generally have their own monitoring systems, sometimes downloading PAS data into an off-the-shelf database package (or an EIS), sometimes entering PAS-generated reports into spreadsheet packages by hand. Whichever method is used they generate information that monitors each separate contract rather than each directorate's (or trust's) caseload as a whole.

Access to information

It should be possible for other NHS managers to arrange with the information manager a routine, say monthly, information pack that details the activity taking place in any individual area of interest. Care should be taken in the choice and depth of material requested – it is easy to be overwhelmed with oceans of virtually useless printouts each month. No single suite of data or information will satisfy all needs so one cannot draw up definitive lists for every imaginable directorate or department. However a few basic rules begin the process of getting the right information to the right place at the right time.

The first is: consult the local information team. Its members know what types of data are held where, how to access them, and how to produce information from them. A second rule is: be prepared to discuss requirements. The information team will probably not know in advance precisely what information a particular manager needs (and probably he or she won't either). An indication of managerial objectives will be required to begin the information ball rolling. It is easy to fall into the 'information trap':

'I need some information',
'What sort of information?',
'Well, what sorts have you got?'
'Lots of different types, what do you need?',
'I'm not sure, but I know I need some information.'
(compare Welch 1993: 15)

Relatively concise managerial objectives should be apparent from the relevant business plan, and it is as well to remember that information staff are there not only to access data but also to advise on suitable data items and analyses. It is also necessary to decide what data or information are critical to running the business and therefore to monitor regularly. It should not be necessary to have every single detail of activity delivered every month in a wheelbarrow full of paper. The higher the organisation level, the less detail required, the easier to produce the monitoring information, and the easier it is to monitor the business. The trick is both to decide what is crucial for 'fast glance' monitoring, and to ensure that identified problems can be easily delved into in order to get to the various levels of detail as required.

The contents of any information pack should be agreed between the manager and the information team. The agreement should be flexible in order to cater for unforeseen future needs (which are likely). The pack should consist of statistical, graphical and textual information and should cover activity, financial and manpower data. These packs will probably consist of fairly broad overviews and be paper based; if further detail is required, a separate *ad hoc* information request will probably be needed. These usually arise in respect of activity information. If users feel confident with information technology there is nothing to stop managers arranging electronic data downloads (either from floppy discs or over a network) into spreadsheet or database software for analysis at leisure. (It is important to stick to trust-wide standards on software and hardware, though, to ensure sources of advice and support, and to ensure that a thorough knowledge of data structure, standards and meanings is gained before attempting any analysis. See Chapter 1.)

Access through a HISS interface or a CMMS terminal or PC has an enormous advantage over the more traditional paper-based information pack environment. A suite of self-defined reports with accompanying graphics chosen from a personal menu can be accessed. These can be set up by the information team and activated by personal password. After training in information management and technology (IM&T) many further queries can be answered by either 'drilling down' to the next level of data, or by utilising one of the flexible and sensitive report-writing tools that invariably accompanies modern equipment. Unfortunately, most NHS hospitals survive on data collection systems that are not geared to flexible and easy information access. Probably paper-based information packs will be the first port of call for most managers.

Information packs

With so many information sources in the NHS, the myriad 'businesses' and the variety of methods for accessing, analysing and delivering information, it would be too Herculean a task for the present writer to prescribe information pack contents for every conceivable use. However, as a general working example that might be modified for other areas, let us examine the possible routine information needs of a typical surgical directorate in a district general hospital catering for general surgery, ENT, urology, oral surgery and ophthalmology. Theatres do not come within the direct control of this particular directorate.

It is advisable to have routine information delivered at least monthly; and to stick to 'high-level' views for most routine needs, investigating any trouble-spots by *ad hoc* requests for more detail in the relevant area. Any routine information pack should have a first page that serves as a 'map' for succeeding pages; this will probably be graphical and indicate in 'fast-glance' fashion the condition of the directorate. Information should be offered on activity (number of inpatients treated, including day cases), outpatients (new attenders or total), budget position and manpower variations. Arranged for clarity at a glance (as opposed to wading through tomes of dusty data), graphs should show the directorate's budgetary position, manpower use (including use of bank staff) and caseload – all noting variance from the planned baselines. The baseline must, of course, have taken into account any planned increases (set in the business plan and based on historical data with seasonalised projections). The next page(s) should 'drill down' to the next level of information – in this case splitting the directorate into its specialities; and within speciality into its consultant firms. Other pertinent fast-glance indicators such as waiting list position, proportion of day case work carried out, average length of episodes and bed occupancy can be added to the slightly more detailed data.

The layout of the data pack should be quite deliberate. It should represent a logical path from high-level view down to reasonably detail. The first level of detail will show the position of the directorate for the year so far; succeeding pages should give a detailed month-by-month account of performance. The more detailed pages should indicate how many beds on average were available to each speciality and how many were occupied (note that bed occupancy is counted at midnight and does not necessarily reflect bed use during the day). These data represent the first building blocks of any local indicators (see below). The next items should deal with inpatient workload, split between elective and non-elective cases and compared to the plan. This is important. In attempting to influence the directorate's caseload pattern, the manager can normally only influence the number of elective patients (those drawn from waiting lists, including day case work). Non-elective patients tend to arrive in unplanned fashion. Outpatient caseload can also be planned (though special arrangements might be necessary for collecting pertinent information). The manager might bear in mind the relative costs of inpatient, day case and outpatient work (and their relative impact on bed and ward resources) and consider shifting some inpatient work onto a day case basis and some day case work to outpatients. *A Short Cut to Better Services* (Audit Commission 1990) recommends 20 day case procedures. The information team might help model the potential changes.

The next page(s) of the data pack should be devoted to standard local indicators derived from the aforementioned base data. These include: the proportion of inpatients treated as day cases, the average length of episode (how long a patient is under a particular consultant's care), turnover interval (how long beds are empty), throughput (how many patients have used a particular speciality or directorate bed in the year), and percentage occupancy (how many beds are occupied, on average). These indicators should be placed alongside Regional or national averages to be more managerially useful. Critical scrutiny of these indicators will give a good idea of how heavily beds are being used and may prompt ideas on more efficient bed management (say, converting a seven-day ward to a five-day ward or day case ward). Note, though, that these are merely indicators and no precipitate action should be taken on the basis of this information alone. Rather, they indicate areas for more detailed and sensitive investigation.

It is becoming increasingly important to manage the mix of cases handled by each clinician, for some kinds of cases consume far more resources than others. The right balance between cases with low- and high-resource consumption is necessary for budgetary control. Many trusts will not have a fully functioning CMMS (see above) but it should still be possible to get some indication of case-mix from routinely generated data and to add this to any paper-based, routine information pack. Again it is simpler for the manager to begin with 'high level' case-mix information and send *ad hoc* requests if further details are required. It is best to 'group' cases into meaningful categories. For example, some trusts (and purchasers) find it useful to differentiated GPFH (general practitioner fundholder) funded cases (split into their respective price-bands) from others (see below). This splits the total caseload into five or six bandings. It can then be subdivided by consultant firm, monitored monthly. If the data have been coded it will also be possible to analyse the caseload by DRGs or HRGs (see Chapter 9). These groupings can be augmented; for example, surgical directorates might wish to monitor endoscopic work separately from other cases. Orthopaedic divisions might want to monitor hips and knees separately. Trusts as a whole may wish to monitor numbers of procedures in the Audit Commission's 'basket' of twenty types of day cases. Managers need to decide which particular cases are of interest. These can then be abstracted from PAS data using clinical codes (see Chapter 9), fed to a database, aggregated, assigned to local indicators such as those outlined above and reported in the routine data pack.

On a topical note, high level waiting list data should also be included, together with graphical analyses. Overall waiting list trends will then become immediately discernible and the necessary managerial action can be taken. The more detailed split into consultant firms pinpoints particularly troublesome waiting lists. The answer to reducing waiting lists may not wholly lie in increasing elective admissions; this might only exacerbate any existing 'over-achievement' or 'overheating' (a dilemma currently facing many NHS professionals). Waiting list information may, however, prompt a waiting list review in which all patients waiting, say, over six months are contacted to ascertain whether they wish to remain on the list (the number who do not, for one reason or another, can be surprising). At the same time, it should be possible to analyse each list by diagnosis and/or proposed operation to determine how many people might be treated as outpatients (many patients actually prefer a 'swift in and out' treatment to spending time in a hospital bed), or even how many patients might be treated in a primary healthcare setting rather than hospital. In these ways waiting lists might be reduced without inflating elective inpatient and day case caseloads. They also show the value of routine, accurate and timely waiting list information.

While outpatient work consumes far fewer resources per head than in-patient work, far more hospital attendances take place in clinics than on wards and far more outpatient surgical procedures are taking place than ever before. So summary information on outpatient workload should also be included in the monthly information pack. A glance at the graphical first page of the pack should indicate whether a more detailed look at outpatient activity is required. In succeeding pages the data should be split by speciality and consultant and contain standard, basic data items. First, the pack should indicate how many clinics took place and how many were cancelled (the number of cancelled clinics is often a bone of contention; a split by consultant will indicate if any firm needs monitoring). Next, should come details of patient attendances (and of failures to attend). (Information staff refer to 'new' patients as 'referral attendances' and to 'return attendances' as 'consultant initiated'.) Planned numbers and any variances should be among the data. 'Did not attend' (DNA) rates can make interesting reading. It may be useful to establish what sorts of people fail to attend (clearly a larger proportion of those who have been to clinic before than those who are visiting for the first time) and whether it is appropriate to issue multiple appointments to these sorts of people in the first place. In the drive to allocate individual appointment slots it may be wasteful to have large numbers of people failing to arrive for appointments. Again certain types of cases may be better treated in a primary healthcare setting.

The number of 'GP written requests' should be monitored as an indicator of the demand for the clinic as should the 'number waiting'. As in the inpatients section of the data pack the base data can generate several key local indicators – 'average patients per session' (how busy the clinic is), the 'proportion of new attenders' (indicating how much effort is expended on patients who have attended before) and 'proportion of DNAs' (how many appointments are wasted).

As the NHS moves into the internal market proper there is pressure on directorates to negotiate their own contracts with prospective purchasers. The activity levels will probably be decided on the basis of historical data. The repercussions of over-shooting targets on one contract while under-achieving on another contract depend upon the type of contract and how sensitive the 'trigger mechanism' is. Whilst clinical directors and business managers might see a need to 'slow down' the rate of elective surgery, a blanket approach to this will not be sensitive enough if some contractual targets have not been met. If work for purchaser A is 15 per cent over target and work for purchaser B is 10 per cent under it would clearly be wrong to cut elective surgery across the board. So a regular indication of workload per contract is required (again, at least monthly). This too should consist of a high level view showing caseload per contract (elective and non-elective), OPD procedures if appropriate, and ECR data. Alongside, and fed by the same database, should be the expected and actual income figures, with any variance.

The conjunction of financial data and activity information is often interesting. Many trusts have prices, not for every individual type of case, but for groups of them. The groups may be based on DRGs, HRGs or simple price bands (categories A, B, C, D, like those used by private health services but simpler); or might consist only of those procedures chargeable to GP fundholders (usually on a price per case basis). As each patient is discharged and clinically coded he or she is allocated to a particular price group and contract. The aggregation shows the caseload per contract and the income so generated. In this case the high level view of caseload and income is generated 'from the bottom up' and represents a real joining of financial and activity information. Then it becomes important that directorates take responsibility for ensuring good data quality (if they have managerial control over data input such as coding, admissions, etc.). Bills will be generated on the basis of the collected data. Bad or missing clinical coding will affect the billing process; bad or missing post codes will affect contract allocation; bad or missing GP codes will affect billing to GP fundholders. Remember – no data, no money.

Information concerning quality generally falls into two broad categories: clinical and non-clinical (see Chapter 6). Quality standards are written into most contracts. They often reflect *Patient's Charter* rights (non-clinical information) and whatever local standards have been negotiated. Thus the monthly high-level data pack should also contain indicators on critical standards – re-admission rates, cancelled operations, waiting times in outpatients, length of wait for inpatient treatment, maximum wait for first routine outpatient appointment. These indicators should be graphed over time to pick out any obvious trends and can be broken down further to consultant firms, particular outpatient clinics, etc. Clinical quality is often approached through medical or clinical audit. Apart from the selection of cases to be audited, investigations often involve trawling through case notes by hand rather than computerised interrogation. Here CMMSs come into their own – audit through care profiles offers a less labour intensive method of monitoring clinical quality. Care profiles by themselves do not replace full-scale clinical audit but they may become a useful monitoring tool, especially in a contracting context.

As purchasers become more powerful within the internal market, quality issues will become more important. Quality targets, non-clinical as well as clinical, will be written into contracts and contracts may be withdrawn if they are not met. 'League tables' of the sort recently introduced for schools have been established for hospitals, and trusts' scores consist partly of quality measurements – waiting times in outpatients, assessment times in A&E, waiting times for inpatient appointment, cancelled operations and number waiting for selected procedures. Again, it is well worth consulting the local information team to help set up any additional data gathering mechanism.

Directorates may also seek to expand their services – either to increase throughput or offer new services. For marketing a directorate's or trust's services it becomes necessary to analyse the market (see also Chapters 6 and 12). A first decision is just what comprises the trust's or directorate's market. Traditionally, this was expressed as the HA's resident population. It is possible to discover where residents go for treatment. It is reasonably simple to find how many residents attended for a particular treatment and at which hospital; and not difficult to quantify elective and non-elective cases. These data should be presented as a time-series (say, the last five years) to get a firm grasp on growth (or shrinkage) in any particular area. Generally, it will not be possible to affect the destination of acute non-elective attendances; the numbers appearing as elective cases, though, might be considered as potential directorate customers and it is to these people (or rather, to their GPs or HAs) that marketing advances should be made.

Local HA residents, though, may well not form the entire market of the trust. The trust, department or directorate may routinely treat numerous people from outside the HA boundary or even the region. This all depends upon the siting of the trust and the services on offer. If this 'cross-boundary flow' occurs regularly, other authorities' residents are part of the trust's market. The interesting problem for information specialists is how to obtain useful information on other District's residents – and, harder still, on other regions' residents – and then to decide how much of that district or region is a potential market. These sorts of data will probably not automatically be available to managers in each monthly information pack but tend to be serviced by *ad hoc* requests for information (see Chapters 6 and 12). They are a good example of the sort of *ad hoc* query that can be fired at information teams, queries restricted only by the questioner's imagination and the databases' interface capabilities.

There is no need for general or clinical managers to be highly computer literate information specialists: the local information manager is there not only to process requests for information and to analyse that information, but to advise upon it as well. A monthly data-pack arranged as described above should meet most activity monitoring needs. If there are further details needed managers should never be afraid to ask the information team – they are there to help and if they can't, they probably know a man who can.

Data quality – the role of doctors, nurses and managers

The Resource Management Initiative (RMI) consisted of two major thrusts: getting clinical staff more involved in the managerial aspects of healthcare; and providing better information to assist in that. The CMMS was seen as the central tool for enhancing the provision of information at trust level. As lessons emerged from the initiative and it was extended to other trusts, it became clear that while the initiative devolved access to data (away from the central information team, towards general, clinical and directorate managers) little was done about devolving responsibility for data quality.

As directorates begin to take over roles previously held by a central team (clinical coding, medical records, direct input of data to PAS, etc.) so they must also accept responsibility for the quality of data generated. A well-known saying in computing circles is: 'Rubbish in – rubbish out'. If the quality of data put into a computer is poor, the quality of information coming out is corresponding poor, regardless of the operators' skills or the size and complexity of the computer. If managers are to rely upon information routinely generated by trust systems, they must also be able to rely upon the quality of that information. If they are to believe the generated information, the more they personally 'own' it, the better. In theory the development of directorates should give their staff greater local control over input, hence greater the local 'ownership', better quality of input, and more credible information.

Some health workers, among them clinicians, tend to be skeptical of current information offerings. How can doctors, nurses and therapists be brought into the information world? In many ways, of course, they will have to get involved as their managerial responsibilities increase as resource management continues. Realistically, though, it is only through direct involvement in the collection of data that clinicians can achieve any sense of ownership. Many doctors are becoming involved in clinical coding, in costing and pricing for certain procedures, and in ensuring that their caseloads are correctly and completely recorded on the information system. Nurse management information systems (NMIS) are becoming more common (as an adjunct to the resource management project CMMS). Data on paramedical therapies is increasingly in demand, especially by GP fundholders, and so systems of information gathering in these areas are also under the microscope.

Devolving the responsibility for data collection to the directorates has a direct impact upon the central information team. General, clinical and directorate managers who are not experienced at managing data and information require training. Few people have this experience, and even fewer trainers. One pool of available expertise is, of course, the local information team. The deeper one moves into the HISS and resource management the clearer it becomes that a training exercise of truly gigantic proportions is required within most trusts. This training exercise must be in at least three parts. One covers IT – what is a computer, how to use PC software, how to use the current applicants (PAS, radiology, pathology, etc.). A second includes data definition training (just what is a day case, a bed, an operative procedure?); and the third should centre on how to use these data items to produce information for business use. In short, managers need to be trained in the tools they can use, in the shape of the building blocks, and in exactly what they can build with them. A start has been made with the recent launch of the NHS information management and technology strategy (see Chapter 2) and information-centred courses within various university departments. However, much in-house training continues to be focused more around how to use PCs and their associated software rather than what they are being used for in the first place.

Changes unleased by Resource Management, *Working for Patients* (Department of Health 1989a), *Community Care Agenda for Action* (Department of Health 1988) and the *Patient's Charter* have demanded volumes of information hitherto unknown. By and large NHS information systems, historically under-funded and under-valued, have responded sluggishly. Nevertheless, some progress has been made following the examples set by the RMI and HISS pilot sites. More important, perhaps, has been the re-orientating of trust information teams away from dealing almost solely with the requirements of the centre to understanding and responding to the demands of in-house 'businesses'. Here lies yet another challenge for the local information team. Not only must specialist information workers be willing to accept the use of information systems by non-specialists. In any event, but especially in the absence of suitable in-house training schemes, it is to the local information team that trust managers should turn for discussion of information needs, analyses and pointers to interpretation. The level of service enjoyed by general, clinical and directorate managers within trusts – not to mention the level of service experienced by patients themselves – will depend largely upon how far and how well local information teams have progressed with this re-orientation.

Chapter 6

INFORMATION FOR QUALITY ASSURANCE

Rod Sheaff

Managing service quality at provider level

In an NHS trust or other commercialised healthcare provider, the strategy for managing service quality, and hence the supporting information systems, are necessarily part of the trust's wider marketing activity. NHS policy documents suggest that when trusts negotiate with purchasers service quality should be an important selling point (Department of Health 1989: 22, 35). In doing so, trusts have two main strategy options.

A minimal strategy is to show that trust services satisfy respectable minimum (or slightly higher) quality and safety standards; for instance that the trust passes 'organisational audit' (accreditation), has BS5750 or ISO9000 recognition or participates in national quality control systems. For this, its information systems must both satisfy the accreditors (whose requirements are usually documented at length - see below) and generate whatever substantive data they routinely want. It is still too early to say exactly what these requirements will be in the case of organisational audit in the United Kingdom because systems are still being developed. However it appears US and Australian accreditation practice will be the model for a UK system. Australian and US accreditation systems scrutinise medical records for clinical completeness and use in clinical management and quality control, contemporaneity, legibility and confidentiality, staffing of medical records offices, and, in the Australian case, for the adequacy of hospital library systems. But otherwise they say little about information systems (Australian Council on Hospital Standards, annually; US Joint Commission on Accreditation of Healthcare Organizations, annually).

A maximal strategy would be to furnish evidence that the trust maximises the most important aspects of service quality. This strategy demands trusts to be able to anticipate, through market research, what aspect of service quality impress purchasers favourably. Trust information systems then have to produce information that substantiates (as far as they can) the trust's claim to offer such services.

Deming, Juran and others distinguish the two main tasks which are involved in managing service quality. One is, to set quality specifications; the other, to monitor whether they are realised (Deming 1986; Juran 1993). Information is also becoming a constituent of service quality itself. GPs are becoming more conscious of what patient information they want from hospitals. Fundholders are in a position to demand it. DHAs and consortia demand data to illustrate progress implementing the main political initiatives (*Patient's Charter*, *Health of the Nation*, etc.) and to change their efficiency indices in the required direction.

This chapter explains how the so-called 'quality chain' method can be used to design an information system for these purposes at clinic, department or speciality level in a healthcare provider. Also known as the 'service chain' or 'critical path' method (see below), the quality chain method coordinates the management of service quality (and marketing (Sheaff 1991)), and decisions about patient care, with the development of information systems at the service level. It leads through Peel and Dowling's pre-selection and selection stages of information system design (see Chapter 1) to data flow diagramming and entity life history diagramming (Avison and Fitzgerald 1988: 115–20) as preliminary stages for detailed hardware and software design. Since quality chains can be drawn at any level of detail right down to task analysis level, they can be used for planning the work and information system requirements of a whole department, a directorate, or an individual therapeutic procedure. The term 'quality chain' indicates that the outcome and quality of care is the cumulative result of critical events during it, and that in receiving care patients traverse the internal administrative, professional or organisational boundaries of the healthcare providers. This makes quality chains useful for 'total' quality management in healthcare, correcting the occupationally specific 'functional' approach of much health service planning. Focusing on main events, quality chains focus on the most important information required to manage service quality, enabling a minimal information system to be designed rather than an exhaustive (large and expensive) codification of standards and procedures (in contrast to many approaches, especially in nursing). This makes it easier to revise quality management information systems as healthcare techniques change. Quality chains can also be used to coordinate more localised methods of quality management (e.g. accreditation or 'organisational audit', standard-setting, clinical audit, etc.) around each healthcare 'product line'.

A quality chain maps the process of healthcare from the standpoint of the patient. It is drawn by charting main events in the process of care, especially

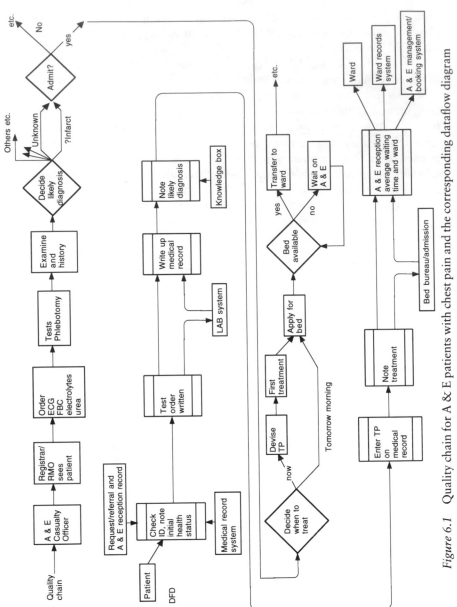

Figure 6.1 Quality chain for A & E patients with chest pain and the corresponding dataflow diagram

the decisions about which referral or treatment options to take, and the criteria by which these decisions are made. For an existing service the chain is first drawn empirically, from direct observation. The top half of Figure 6.1 illustrates a quality chain for accident and emergency patients with chest pains.

One way of drawing a quality chain is from health workers' accounts of how they work. This approach also reveals what events and decision-making criteria they think are clinically pertinent. Parts of the chain may already be documented (e.g. booking, consent, complaints procedures) but how far written procedures are actually followed is another matter. Utilisation studies of referral patterns, screening and detection patterns, self-referral, ambulance referrals, referral bottlenecks, waiting times, charges to patients and DNAs also analyse and explain how patients enter the quality chain and pass along it. Existing information systems may be able to supply some of this (see Chapter 5). Often, however, important parts of a quality chain are not formally recorded at all. Much of the clinical work illustrated in Figure 6.1 is often done by informal routine articulated, as it were, in an oral tradition passed informally from one houseman or registrar to the next.

At the outset one must decide what level of detail to analyse at. One can chart the whole episode of care, a specific event, even a specific intervention (e.g. phlebotomy); logically, the charts corresponding to different levels of generality are nested (Figure 6.2 illustrates for one of the stages in Figure 6.1). One must also define the ends of the chain, which for quality management and marketing purposes may lie outside the hospital or clinic itself. If, for example, one service objective is to attract GP referrals it may be necesary to analyse the relation between general practitioner and outpatient clinic, hence start the quality chain from the patient's consultation with the GP and finish it only with the post-discharge arrangements.

Analysing the quality chain for the purposes of managing service quality, deciding marketing mix, and (then) designing the necessary information system, involves the following steps.

One begins by articulating the objectives of providing the service (the starting point for many methodologies including STRADIS, the varieties of Information Engineering and Multiview (Avison and Fitzgerald 1988: 181–3, 261). It is more necessary to state these frankly and realistically than as a cosmetically attractive 'mission' or similar statement. Service objectives can also be discovered empirically, partly by asking those responsible what criteria their management of the service is actually assessed by, partly by considering the nature of the organisation in which the service stands, and partly by reference to planning and performance review documents. Although commercial and directly publicly managed providers' priorities differ, they will normally cover:

1 Health gain; to maximise the difference between a patient's health status before and after treatment, compared with an alternative treatment or none. Minimally, these objectives imply avoiding iatrogenesis.

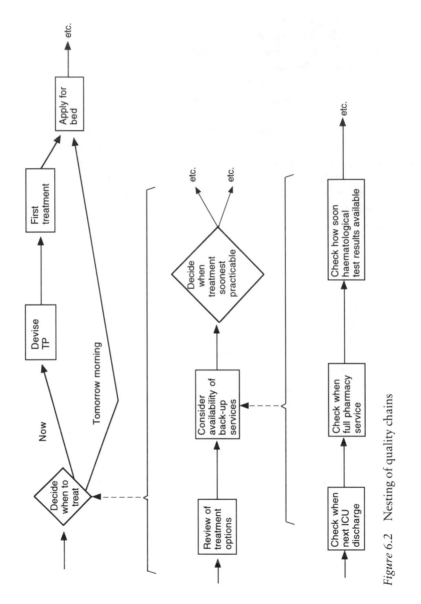

Figure 6.2 Nesting of quality chains

2 Purchaser satisfaction and willingness to repeat contracts (or budgets) and to reimburse work fully.
3 User satisfaction, 'users' taken broadly to include GPs and informal carers besides patients.
4 Third party demands (e.g. legal requirements or national policy objectives).
5 Profitability or cost containment.

These objectives ground the second step, of identifying the key events in the quality chain. 'Key' events are those which determine (causally) whether the service objectives are met or not. Here too staff opinions are often a good starting point for finding out empirically which events are 'key'. Normally the main types will be:

1 Self-referrals, when people try to enter the sick role. The causes and reasons are identified, described and explained by medical-sociological, epidemiological, aetiological research and by consumer research into patients' health and sickness behaviours, compliance, knowledge of health and self-care (e.g. Parsons (1951), Calnan (1987)).
2 Clinicians' referrals, especially the choice of provider and decisions to refer to high-risk or high-cost services.
3 Major events in carrying out the treatment plan efficaciously (e.g. the choice of therapy, administration of anaesthetics, discharge decisions).
4 Events determining purchasers' willingness to buy (or reimburse). In a commercialised setting these include events which attract profitable and repel unprofitable referrals ('skimming' and 'dumping', in US parlance), and events which can be billed to the purchaser or patient as a chargeable 'extra'. (NHS hospitals can only do this within central policy limitations (Waldegrave 1991)). (Timeliness and quality of information itself may be among these key events).
5 Cash flow events: the information system contributes to the quality of financial management by recording referrals; identifying, billing and chasing-up the purchaser; and to service management by preventing service breakdowns that incur financial penalties.

Ranking these key points according to how important the objective they serve is, and how much each event influences whether service objectives are achieved, suggests priorities for the managing service quality and for developing the corresponding information systems.

Next, normative quality standards for the key events are set. A mixture of user-led and provider-led standards is normally necessary. What source is relevant to setting each quality standard depends on the provider's objectives and on the nature of the key event which the standard governs. To attract referrals, the quality standards which a provider has to offer to attract the mix of self-referrals it wants are 'read off' from market research into patients',

GPs' or informal carers' preferences and aversions in service provision. The present provider's services are compared with what patients perceive as the available alternative providers and their corresponding benefits (or defects). For critical treatment events the quality standards are discovered through technical evaluations (clinical trials), treatment protocols, comparative studies, 'benchmark' reports of good practice, clinical standard-setting and (not least) clinical audit. To attract purchasers, providers have again to set quality standards which are relevant to purchasers' requirements, and pitched at a level bearing comparison with substitute providers (e.g. waiting times which are no worse than the main competitors'). For publicly funded purchasers these requirements will normally include meeting national health policy objectives or standards (e.g. *Patients' Charter*) and for accreditation, licensing or registration (with the concommitant quality standards). Standards governing financial management are set partly by the provider's management systems, partly by purchasers' requirements (e.g. for documentation and monitoring information), and partly by what events trigger bonus or penalty payments under the service contracts. Finding indicators by which to operationalise and monitor these key quality standards is sometimes simple (referral numbers, numbers of pounds, nationally stipulated monitoring indicators, waiting times in minutes etc.) but sometimes very difficult (e.g. for clinical outcomes, although some critical catalogues of health status and outcome indicators are becoming available (e.g. Bowling 1991; Wilkin *et al.* 1992)).

A more thorough modernisation of a service, or the design of a new service, can be made by reconstructing its quality chain from scratch. Depending on the case, it may be possible to remove or simplify steps (e.g. to eliminate intermediate waiting areas by introducing individual appointment times in an outpatients department), to innovate new elements (e.g. a triage nurse at the entrance to an accident and emergency department) or new methods of performing existing activities (e.g. keyhole instead of traditional surgery).

Either way, the resulting standards have often to be moderated in practice by considerations of feasibility or implementation, especially their acceptability to influential bodies such as the provider's own medical establishment. Implementing new quality standards is no small task, although beyond the remit of a book on informatics (see Øvretveit 1991, Sheaff 1991).

Once available, the quality chain analysis indicates concretely what sort of information system is required for managing service quality. How this is done, we next consider.

Provider 'intelligence' level

Setting the substantive quality standards for an NHS trust, or similar commercialised, service demands five main types of information. The preceding section listed these as information about the trust's specific objectives; about the health system context within which it works; about users' preferences in regard to service quality; about current best practice, in terms of service quality; and about the 'key events' which determine what quality of service is actually achieved. An information system about these matters can only be only partly automated, because so much of this information is amorphous, informal, qualitative and verbal. For example, insofar as service objectives are recorded, it will exist in documentary form as business plans, policy statements (ELs (executive letters), HCs (health circulars), etc.), 'mission statements' and the like (see Rea: 1993). It is partly informal and unstructured, and the system for collecting this information consists of a set of managerial and clinical networks. This largely qualitative part of the information system is sometimes called the 'intelligence' level (Atkinson 1992: 6). This section considers what information and what information systems it demands.

Quality chain analysis can reveal how much of this information already exists informally: what information staff already use for setting quality standards (which they will not necessarily articulate as such) at the critical events and where they obtain it (Greenhalgh & Co. 1992). Objectives for the service have to be articulated to get the management of quality started at all. At service level, the objectives of most immediate practical importance are printed in service contracts. In many instances important provider or policy objectives will not be written down at all, or written in broad, vague terms. Interpretation is necessary to establish what objectives such as 'cost effectiveness' are to be taken to mean, or what the purchasers were actually trying to influence or stipulate when they negotiated or let the service contract.

Where NHS services compete, a market analysis is necessary to establish which are the main local substitute services against which the trust's own service quality must bear comparison. Chapter 12 considers what this involves at trust level. For each service, trust information systems will have to furnish comparitor data about competitors' quality strengths and weaknesses, for 'competitive benchmarking' of the quality of the trust's services against these competitors. The Welsh NHS is adopting national benchmarking. A database of best norms of service quality and practice serves as an open reference point against which providers (and purchasers) can check a particular provider's own quality standards. The market analysis would also have to catalogue the main local purchasers (DHAs or geographical consortia, GP fundholders, local authorities, private patients and other private purchasers), noting for each what service quality characteristics these purchasers particularly value (and disvalue). These will include national quality standards such as *Patients' Charter* standards on waiting times. Behavioural and administrative data on patient flows, expecially cross-boundary flows, provide clues about this. This shows which aspects of service quality (e.g. access times, availability of day surgery) it is necessary for management information systems to concentrate on in presenting data on service quality to purchasers for service contracting purposes. The market analysis would also identify any incipient changes in the 'technology' of the service in question: new models of care, new types of treatment, and new ways of substituting primary for hospital care, or outpatient for inpatient care. Background social and epidemiological trends likely to influence the trust's patient flows and case mix, or expose gaps and duplications of the trust's services are also necessary. All this analysis ought to occur for business planning purposes at trust level anyway, but managers responsible for service quality will need access to those parts of it relevant to their services. Few trusts yet undertake these analyses.

Similarly, an intelligence level information system for setting quality standards has to summarise users' views on what aspects of service quality are important to them, hence what the corresponding service quality standards ought to be. (Whether the trust can or would wish to provide services of this quality is another matter. If managers decide not to, the corollary of a quality strategy is a promotional strategy to explain to users why the trust is providing the kind of service it does.) Here service 'users' include not only patients but informal carers, GPs, and voluntary bodies, both charities and special interest or pressure groups (such as Shelter). All this necessitates collecting three types of data: existing data on user preferences and behaviour; qualitative information of the sort generated in the types of local consultation that *Local Voices* recommends (Department of Health 1991); and new, tailored market research data to meet whatever gaps remain. To the quality indicators which users identify a trust can add indicators for monitoring its own marketing innovations. An example is Homewood Trust's policy of checking that a wreath is sent on the trust's behalf to patients' funerals.

Collecting existing data on user preferences or behaviour may, to a limited extent, be automatable through database searches and re-analysing PAS data (see Chapter 5) but will largely consist of manual collation such as taking local press-cuttings. New primary market research can be done either by the trust's own staff or bought in, but either way the research has to be so managed and designed that the trust's information systems retain the primary data for future and different re-analyses. The 'intelligence' system has to be able to support the routine generation of questionnaires and other data-collection methods, the actual data collection, entry and analysis (cf. Luck *et al.* 1988; Chisnall, 1991). What indicators are used for those aspects of service quality where the patient is the best or only judge (e.g. whether they felt they received adequate explanation of their condition, could find their way round the hospital, etc.) will vary from trust to trust. Even if standard indicators of such factors as staff politeness could be developed, few are available yet.

For quality standards which are set internally on a technical basis, the information system has to contain means of generating normative 'bench-marks'. One way is to take best internally achieved clinical practice as the quality standard. Many hospitals in effect do this by comparing per-consultant figures for such indicators as length of stay for each main type of case. Then the clinicians themselves begin generating and levelling up their own practice standards (Buxton *et al.* 1991). Clinical audit systems and ready-made standard-setting packages (e.g. a checklist grid such as Wilson's (1993) are two other ways. Alternatively, quality standards may be generated through accreditation systems. Acquiring BS5750 or ISO9000 registration largely depends on demonstrating that systems – in essence, information systems – exist for deriving quality standards, checking that the service actually conforms, and documenting all this (Rooney 1988). For treatment protocols the Strategic Intent and Direction (SID) system can be used in a similar way (Welsh Office NHS Directorate 1990a). Other clinical and research databases can be used in a similar way, including national benchmarking centres such as the Welsh one.

If health gain is the fundamental criterion of service quality, the most important indicators of service quality are outcome indicators. The intelli-gence level of a quality information system has therefore to discover and select suitable outcome indicators. Even a small trust requires a variety of quality indicators, possibly selecting different indicators for reporting to different purchasers' requirements. One possibility would be for providers and purchasers to chose quality indicators for each service contract from a national database of validated quality indicators used for benchmarking centres or in clinical databases. Proprietary clinical management and risk-management systems, especially of US provenance, are sometimes sold with clinical indicators built in (e.g. an index for severity of patient's condition on admission). A few outcome indicators will be stipulated by the purchasers or by national policy, or implied by law (e.g. deaths during surgery). A service can also generate its own, 'clinically pertinent' indicators through formalising the indicators that clinicians already implicitly use (often informally, unarticulated and unrecorded). Clinical audit is one way of doing this. Published directories and guides to outcome indicators are also appearing (Bowling 1991; Wilkins *et al.* 1992; Department of Health, annually) and databases are being established in Leeds and Manchester. The technical complexity of devising new outcome indicators should not be underestimated. It is a research and development task in itself. (Bowling (1991: 1–22) and Holland (1983) indicate some areas of difficulty.) Mana-gerially useful indicators are standardly defined and, if necessary, standardi-sable (to enable comparisons between services and consultant teams); and deal with aspects of health status (e.g. restoration of function, pain control, morale and mental state, self-care and health maintenance) which are meaningful to patients and clinicians.

According to the quality chain method, the 'key' service events are those for which it is most necessary to set and monitor quality standards. What some of the key events are, will either be fairly self-evident or will be stipulated in service contracts and in policy documents such as *Patients' Charter*. Others are less obvious and one task of the intelligence level of the information system is to reveal them. A recently discovered example is the relationship between the volume of cases of a specific clinical type that a clinician handles and the outcome he or she achieves. There are two main ways an information system can collect data identifying key events. One is by accessing existing clinical research databases. Another is by analysing past service data for correlations between quality indicators and other factors such as case mix, type of treatment, referral route, clinical 'firm' and so on. Such correlations have then to be investigated further to find whether they indicate a causal relationship. Cumulative monitoring data can also be used for analysing causal relations between key service events and the provider's objectives, hence evaluating what impacts new working methods have on service quality.

This obviously requires a monitoring system capable of accumulating past data on how well the service has performed against its quality standards at the key events. Once the intelligence level of the information system is in place, construction of this level of the quality monitoring information system can proceed.

Monitoring level

One purpose of an information system for monitoring service quality is to check that the quality standards are being realised. Others are to provide data for diagnosing quality shortfalls to prevent recurrence; to generate data on service quality for use in managing service contracts; for public relations and promotional uses; and for reporting to higher bodies. Having determined what quality standards to work to, the next step is to derive from the quality chain a grid-based specification of the information system and a data flow diagram (DFD). DFDs are the basis for several information systems methodologies, e.g. STRARDIS (Gane and Sarson 1979), Information Engineering, Structure and Systems Analysis and Design and the tasks described below are comparable to steps 1 to 3 of SSADM methodology (Avison and Fitzgerald 1988: 197). Mapping DFDs from the quality chain is similar to the making of A-graphs in the ISAC (Information System Work and Analysis of Changes) methodology (Avison and Fitzgerald 1988: 216–30). The point of using a quality chain approach to derive the DFD is to ensure the DFD reflects service managers' and clinicians' actual information needs. Using the grid and DFD software and hardware can be selected (see Chapter 11).

Following the patient's progress along the quality chain one notes each point where data are captured or used. They indicate at which event:

1 Each new datum can be input.
2 Data will have to be imported from other systems, e.g. from the PAS or financial systems for costing or billing (see Chapter 5).
3 Data already captured or imported will be used again.
4 Order entries for supplies or support services (laboratories, blood, ambulance, etc.) will be necessary.
5 The quality monitoring system will have to upload summary reporting data into (organisationally) higher-level management information systems.
6 Dedicated clinical or technical systems are required, e.g. to control complex equipment such as scanners.

Junctions in the quality chain indicate the main patient management decisions, hence the people and decisions which require management (including clinical management) information system outputs. The description of these decision points in the quality chain chart indicates who should receive what information about which key events, and how often. What information, hence what data, they require can be inferred from the objectives formulated during the quality chain analysis, and by consulting them (see the previous section). In these ways the networks and dataflows of both patient administration system and management information system can be charted, and related to dedicated clinical or technical systems (see Figure 6.1). Points at which data have to be collected and used show where the information system users' terminals have to be. For each of these a grid like that in Table 6.1 can be used to collate decisions about what data to collect, analyse and report. Listed on the vertical edge of the table, these decisions concern:

1 what quality indicators to apply to each event
2 what the corresponding datasets are
3 how to capture these data
4 how to analyse and present them
5 who to report the results to
6 access to data, security and confidentiality.

Each column corresponds to a quality chain key event. The six information decisions about each key event have to be consistent with those made for the other key events – another reason for minimising the number of key events to monitor. The grid offers a way to design an information system tailored to a particular service, for considering each aspect of the information system systematically and revealing any scope for simplifying or reducing it. Table 6.1 gives part of a (fictional) grid for the quality chain in Figure 6.1.

What types of indicators are necessary to monitor service quality, and some sources, were briefly noted in the previous section, identifying outcome

Table 6.1   Key service events and information system events

	A&E officer	RMO	Order tests	etc
Quality indicators	Access time, accurate triage	Access time Accurate diagnosis	All and only relevant tests ordered	
Datasets	patient history, vital signs, BP, etc.	Further clinical data	Patient identifier, doctor ordering type of test	
Data capture by Analyses	Houseman collate, compare with clinical audit benchmarks	RMO collate, compare with clinical audit benchmarks	Doctor ordering Collate, tabulate	
Presentation Report to	Run chart Consultant, medical audit	Run chart Consultant, medical audit	Summary tables Pathology director, consultant, clinical directorate	
Access	Consultant, medical audit, patient	Consultant medical audit, patient	Consultant, medical audit, patient, Chief executive officer (anonymised data only)	
Security	Personal password, logged use	Personal password, logged use	Personal password, logged use	
Confidentiality; access limited to	The above or 'need to know' basis only	The above or 'need to know' basis only	The above or 'need to know' basis only	

indicators as the most important and problematic. For evaluating health gain during the episode of care the indicators must be comparable between start and finish of the patient episode. Admission and discharge summaries must therefore record (among other things) a common set of health status indicators (see below).

The choice of quality indicators (see the previous section) determines what datasets to collect. Some indicators only require a single data item (e.g. a vision or severity score), while others require many (e.g. SIP, Nottingham Health Profile). Partly the choice of datasets depends on what methods are used for managing the quality of clinical work. Clinical audit and risk management both demand the scrutiny of patient records which record predetermined categories of event (e.g. unplanned readmission, formal complaint). For risk management, indicators of untoward events must be included, with a view to relating these to other quality and clinical data and as an early warning system for handling claims and preventing recurrences

(Lingren 1992). Clinical audit usually requires random selection of patient histories, making an identifier of each health record (whether or not this is the patient identifier) an indispensible data item. In any event, a basic PAS dataset (name, NHS number, date of birth, address) has to be linked to the other datasets for the same patient. Table 6.1 simply lists the dataset items under each heading. Each data item will require its own definitions, preferably industry, national or international standard definitions. One way to achieve this is by linking the information system to an on-line data dictionary, which can also stipulate acceptable formats and value-ranges for each data set (Health Information Strategy Steering Group 1991: 7, 18). Various techniques exist for checking the completeness of data sets and the logical relations within them (Gane and Sarson 1979: ch. 4, give examples). Here a generalist is probably wise to seek specialist help.

The quality chain indicates when occurrent data can be captured during the patient episode and by whom. Data on health status and patient events are recorded by clinicians and administrators in the course of writing the individual patient record and entering orders. Earlier sections suggest that it will be necessary to supplement these data, for quality management purposes, by importing data from elsewhere in the trust, from external databases and from market research. Data can often be imported from other trust information systems such as a THIS or order entry system, or from the PAS or GP's system to generate a new patient record or re-open an existing one once a few patient identifiers (name, address, date of birth and other identifiers) are known (see Chapter 4). Table 6.1 also has a line noting how data will be captured; 'capture' includes not only the data sources but also any necessary methods of data verification.

During the patient episode the individual patient record is (or should be, by English law) the repository for all data used to evaluate the patient's health and for clinical management. Since data should be collected once only and since management information systems should use routinely collected data wherever possible, this suggests that a longitudinal individual patient record should become the main source of data about the patient episode (as in intended for CISP; see Bullas et al. 1993: 49). This is as much a matter of developing the medical record to make it a suitable source of data as of exploiting data that medical records already hold (see Chapter 8). Two implications are relevant here. Formal health status indicators should, first, be a standard data field in the medical record (which indicators are used will depend on the factors discussed in the previous section). The word 'formal' is used to indicate standard, structured indicators as opposed to ad hoc notes of signs and symptoms (which serve different purposes) or data about biological or biochemical systems (which are not necessarily informative about health status at the level of a patient's functioning, pain or morale). To evaluate health gain it is, secondly, necessary to record each patient's health status at least at the start of the episode of care and at the finish. This already happens in some specialities, for instance in vision testing before and after many ophthalmological treatments. Ideally, the last data on the health status of patients who survive would be recorded just when the full effects of treatment had worked through, either at follow-up clinics or by GPs or community health services who would then copy them to the secondary provider. In practice, however, trust information systems will generally have to treat the start and finish of the episode of care admission (by referral or self-referral) and discharge or death respectively.

Quality chain analysis identifies key events in the patient episode, selects quality indicators for them and formulates their target levels. The fundamental analysis is therefore to compare the actually achieved quality indicator levels for each key event. Often quite simple analyses are of greatest practical use; knowing who is referring patients and who is not, the distributions of length of stay, simple outcome measures (such as unplanned readmissions) and so on. For many management purposes it will be enough to analyse the quality data distributions by service contract, directorate, consultant, budget-head, speciality and GP. More complex analyses are easy to automate using modern software, to indicate what mean or mode figures for length of stay, waiting time and other main quality indicators. Comparisons across different clinicians, directorates and departments presuppose at least some common indicators of service quality (hence standardised nosologies, Benson 1991: 71).

Accumulated past data enable current figures to be compared with medium-term trends, to reveal whether changes over the last reporting period are within the normal range of fluctuations or whether they indicate a more significant change. Analyses of data distributions can be used to distinguish isolated quality failures (by accident or individual incompetence) from failures which display a statistical regularity through faulty design of the quality chain or persistent under-resourcing or mismanagement. At this point the information can start to reveal matters demanding practical attention. Figure 6.3 illustrates some commonly seen presentations with possible interpretations.

Quality indicators and statistical process control make it possible to stipulate 'trigger levels' of the indicators of key events so that the system automatically notifies relevant clinicians or managers when a quality indicator falls below that level. By combining clinical protocols with computerised individual patient records systems could be developed to notify the clinician automatically of deviations from treatment protocols or from the expected outcome. Already some proprietary clinical information systems automatically report deviant clinical events or test results to their users. In order to prevent errors rather than detect them after the event, a probable future development using similar principles is automated decision support for clinicians. Such systems link data on key clinical variables in the quality chain with reports from knowledge-based expert systems (WHO

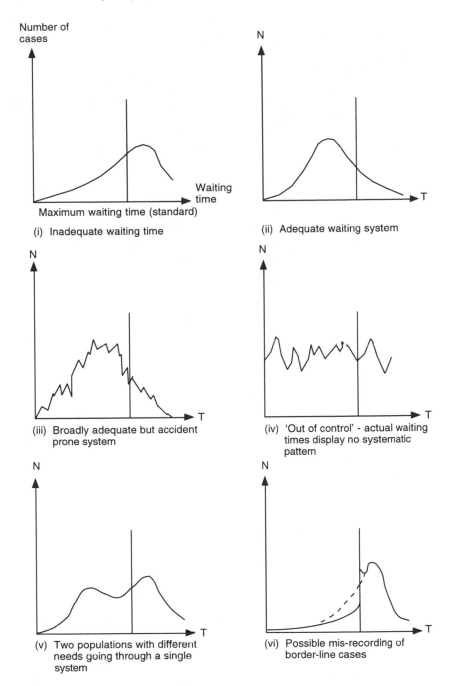

Figure 6.3 Quality indicators and statistical process control – examples of common forms

1988: 54f). This enables clinicians to apply an expert knowledge base to their own working data. Early systems of this type have shown promising results (see De Dombal *et al.* 1972).

Many texts on statistical process control explain these methods (Deming 1986), whose principles have been known for fifty years. What is new, is that policy, financial and competitive pressures are bringing these methods forcibly to the attention of health service managers.

The main principle in deciding reporting arrangements is to ensure that information (analysed and presented data) reaches all those who need to use it for decision making, in time for them to use it. For example, analyses of changes in case mix need to reach (say) nurse managers in time for them to adjust nursing rosters. The use of 'triggers' for automatic reporting has already been mentioned. Similarly, information systems can be used to support clinical audit by randomly selecting patient notes for audit, automatically extracting relevant data and anonymising the notes. The RCS, for instance, already publish advice on automating clinical audit (RCS 1991). An often-neglected reporting route is to patients. McDougall and Brittain (1992: 10,18–9) suggest patients might have access to information on the following aspects of service quality: how to refer themselves to self-help projects, data on waiting lists and times, information on common diseases (presented in lay terms, with information about how to access more technical details in databases for patients who wish), guidance on self-care, and access to foreign-language translations of the foregoing.

The 'Security' line on Table 6.1 prompts a decision on how access to data will be controlled. Passwords are one means; another is a 'filter' to remove patient and clinician identifiers when cases are selected for clinical audit, for risk management purposes, or to investigate an 'untoward incident'. Commercialised providers have also to consider the commercial confidentiality of quality data, beyond that which they are contracted to supply to the purchasers, as a source of competitive advantage. Third parties, such as the Home Office registration of domestic accidents or NAI registers, also have a statutory claim on some data. Methods such as an immediate data access diagram (Gane and Sarson 1979: 95) can be used to chart graphically who needs access to what data. The NHSME information strategy proposes that installation of the security systems should be followed up with small systems reviews and, on large systems, risk analyses (NHSME-IMG 1993b). To confirm the security of data there must be the necessary systems with correct documentation, for instance complete and reliable audit trails to verify that only bona fide users have access to the data. When information is used for commercial purposes obvious doubts arise about its veracity and completeness. This places a premium on using data collected by a disinterested third party where possible, or failing that giving purchasers the opportunity to verify the accuracy and completeness of data and information presented.

Another aspect of security is security of the whole information system and of the patient services which depend on it. In designing an automated information system one should always remember that one day it will fail, and have a contingency plan ready for the failure (see Seabrook 1993). Five safeguards are to:

1 Have a written contingency plan anticipating what to do when the information system crashes, including identifying a backup source of information and services.
2 Ensure top managers scrutinise this plan in detail, and participate in writing it.
3 Review the plan regularly as circumstances change.
4 Train the staff in what the contingency plan requires of them.
5 Check the susceptibility of the information system to industrial action.

The above methods give a first estimate of how many and how large the datasets will be, what data volume and storage are involved, who will require 'real-time' (or 'on-line') access to the system and what outputs are required. From this potential suppliers can begin to estimate what software, networking and hardware will be required. Two strategies for installation then open up. The DFD can be used to guide the design of a bespoke system; or as a guide for buying proprietary hardware and software which construct a system corresponding to the DFD. Chapter 11 explores these questions further and some implementation issues are addressed next.

Chapter 7

IMPLEMENTING AN INFORMATION STRATEGY AT LOCAL LEVEL

Simon Aldridge

Information systems in organisations

This chapter discusses methods of implementing information systems at a local level, illustrating the need to use information systems in a managerial and organisational context. Information and the technology systems are not a end in themselves but are an increasingly important tool for managers working in an ever more complex healthcare organisation. To be useful to managers, information systems have to be implemented in a manner which is sympathetic to issues which are specific to the organisational situation where they will be used. Introducing information systems is a major change process and should be treated as such, rather than as a purely technical issue.

Information systems are increasingly important to NHS management. This has been reflected in the past two decades as healthcare organisations have moved towards greater use of computerised information systems as their work has grown increasingly complex and management need to make more effective decisions more quickly (Ferlie and McKee 1988; Weiner *et al.* 1986) and introduce a diverse range of systems (Fitter 1987a); from the operational, which simply describe what is happening such as the Körner systems, to the managerial, such as Resource Management (DHSS 1986) which explicitly attempt to provide managers with intelligence on which to make more meaningful managerial decisions, something which was not evident in the late 1970s and early 1980s as official reports indicated (DHSS 1983; Royal Commission on the NHS 1979).

The increasing complexity in decision making facing NHS managers has also been created by new organisational structures and processes since the early 1980s. The introduction of general management from 1984 helped to create a demand for information which did more than provide crude data on activity (Greenhalgh and Todd 1985; Scrivens 1987). Systems such as Clinical Budgeting (Bourn and Ezzamel 1986a; Coles 1988) and its successor Resource Management (DHSS 1986; Greenhalgh 1986; Perrin 1987) were an indication of the need to develop information systems which were meaningful at a local (department and unit) level. More recently the reforms prompted by *Working for Patients* (Department of Health 1989a) have increased demand for more sophisticated information so that purchasers and providers can manage the demands of the internal market (Culyer *et al.* 1990). The trend for developing more sophisticated information systems which are useful at a local (sub-district) basis will accelerate. Self-governing status for provider units and the GP fundholding mean that NHS organisations now have to justify their current work patterns in financial and qualitative terms. Information is increasingly essential at both strategic and local level.

Despite large investment in information systems in the NHS over the last decade the perceived benefits of these systems have been slow in coming. Recent reports (National Audit Office 1990; Buxton *et al.* 1991) state that many NHS information systems have not yet demonstrated substantial enough benefits to justify the investment. To be successful information systems should repay their investment by providing managerial or operational information which benefits the organisation in terms of improved decision making, information which is easily understood by its recipients and easily accessible. It should be reduced to the smallest possible amount to be meaningful, manageable and easily digested by decision makers (Ackoff 1976; Tricker 1983).

The foregoing criticisms of recent NHS information systems suggest that often this does not occur. There are many possible reasons. First, there may be problems in analysing the information needs of the organisation. Problems may exist in obtaining the right data to transform into information. The information system which is designed may prove to be unpopular with members of the organisation or too much meaningless information may be produced. All these reasons indicate pitfalls which can occur when information systems are introduced into such complex organisations as healthcare providers. Existing managerial, cultural and social aspects of the organisation as well as the behaviour of individuals are all likely to change under the influence of new information and its technology. The implementation of information systems can bring about four major changes.

First, work roles can change with the introduction of new technology and information systems. Like any new technology the introduction of computerised information systems can radically change an individual's role in the organisation (Woodward 1958; Hirschheim 1985a). For example, computerised information systems may require large amounts of data to be collected and fed in. The increase of NHS systems (such as the Körner systems) in the late 1970s and early 1980s made the collection and entry of data a more important part of many individuals' jobs. New technology can also alter the working lives of caring professions, such as nurses, through new organisational procedures (Yates 1983). Information systems may increase the level of stress on individuals, such as computer operators, who may have to work under new conditions associated with that technology (Bock 1982; Fitter 1987b).

One example of health workers whose role changed with the introduction of new technology in healthcare organisations was health visitors. In many early Resource Management (RMI) pilot sites in England this group had to collect their own activity data manually. The data were then put into the developing computer systems by trained clerks. Health visitors perceived that they were doing an increasing amount of what they saw as clerical work collecting data which meant little to them because they never received any meaningful information back. The Resource Management (RMI) experiment was seen by many professionals as a managerial control exercise (Aldridge and Walker 1991; Jackson 1990). Those affected by new technology will not necessarily agree or identify with what could be perceived as the collection of data for purely management purposes (Bourn 1987).

Individuals also resist the new roles developing from new information systems if they perceive their new function as potentially boring or if their current routine is under threat. On the other hand, it must be stressed that an individual's role can become more interesting and varied if an information system is designed to maximise job satisfaction which can lead to an increase in motivation (Mumford 1972).

New information can, secondly, exacerbate organisational tensions. The implementation of new information systems can bring new insights on which more informed decisions can be made. Both access to information (in terms of speed and availability) and the ability to use new information becomes an issue. All the above factors can affect on existing power and political relationships within an organisation. New systems can often destabilise existing organisational relationships making information become a 'battleground' for key parties. This situation is heightened in healthcare organisations because they are highly diffuse, with many professions each with their own set of cultural beliefs (Bourn and Ezzamel 1986b; Freidson 1970). Different interpretations on what is not valid information can coexist so that information can exacerbate an already heightened and tense relationship between groups with different agendas. Where new management information systems have provided detailed financial information in US hospitals there have been examples of increased organisational conflicts between clinicians and management over how the information is used to apportion financial resources (Carper and Litschert 1983; Provan, 1987)

Thirdly, the organisation may not have had an information culture. Often individuals or even whole organisations are unused to handling information or the technology associated with modern information systems. If information has not normally been available within the organisation less effective use is made of it when new information systems provide it. Without an 'information culture' there may exist myths and uncertainties among organisational members about the possibilities or deficiencies of an information system. Expectations may run high while the difficulties in implementing a system compatible with the needs of the organisation may be underestimated. Then when problems occur with the systems, motivation for change, user morale and belief in the information systems may decline providing an unsuitable condition for future change. An organisation also may have difficulty appreciating how information travels around an organisation and the systems and processes required to facilitate that flow.

The NHS has only begun to obtain an 'information culture' since the late 1970s (Scrivens 1985) when information became available normally rather than exceptionally, and began to be appreciated as such by managers and staff. Wright (1985a) suggested that the Körner systems were not fully integrated into NHS organisational structures because managers did not fully understand how to best use this new resource. Many studies have shown how GPs have not realised the true benefits of computerised information systems because they believed computers would hinder the traditional doctor–patient relationship (Anderson *et al.*, 1986; Brownbridge *et al.*, 1985, 1984; Cruickshank, 1984; Pringle, 1985; Royal College of General Practitioners, 1980). Such studies contradict official claims that computers facilitate the doctor–patient relationship through improved administration (DHSS 1985).

The organisational structure may, fourthly, be unable to handle increased information flows. Körner information sets which were introduced into an NHS with few formalised methods of collecting data and distributing information at local or hospital level (Winston 1986). The introduction of information systems may mean that restructuring within the organisation may have to take place. For example new departments may have to be developed which manage the information function. With the increasing devolution of information systems to individual NHS units more and more changes in organisational procedures and the availability and role of key personnel (e.g. information managers) will have to occur.

These four problems in implementing and using information systems are common to all organisations. Healthcare organisations arguably find it harder to implement information systems effectively because:

1 *Professional bodies have influence and are independent of management.*
  Organisations with a high element of professional involvement face the

problem in implementing change that there is a group of people with a large degree of power on whom the organisation is dependent (Larson 1977; Raelin 1985). It has been suggested there is a conflict between 'managerial' world views and 'professional' views of how an organisation should be run (Hall 1985). Clinicians take an important place within the healthcare organisation whether through formal decision-making procedures (Smith 1955) or more informally (Butcher 1970; Rothman *et al.* 1971; Schultz and Harrison 1986; Freidson 1963). When healthcare organisations are public bodies as in Great Britain clinicians can often influence decisions through their ability to 'appeal' to a broader public (Harrison, 1988; Harrison *et al.* 1991; Thompson 1987). These professional groups have to be persuaded of the viability of information systems before they can be fully integrated into decision making about them. This can be especially difficult if the information systems monitor the activity or outcomes of their work and link this to resource allocations. Pollitt *et al.* (1988) have written of the problems of persuading clinicians of the validity of Clinical Budgeting in the early 1980s in the NHS. Managers were unable to 'sell' the idea that information which the Clinical Budgeting system produced would be used in a constructive, meaningful manner, not as an excuse for managers to cut services.

2 *Complex and uncertain problems which are difficult to model effectively for information purposes.* In much of the work undertaken in healthcare organisations there is a problem quantifying activities (Roos *et al.* 1974) or the outcome of that activity (Fottler, 1987). Health economists have been criticised (Ashmore *et al.* 1989; Mulkay *et al.* 1987) for their inability to measure and quantify healthcare outcomes or even many outputs. This complexity poses a serious problem because most information systems are intended to quantify activities accurately. This is a major issue for those designing an information system for health care, and an unavoidable one given the nature of healthcare. It is compounded by the fact that often organisational roles can be confused and uncertain with conflicts between departments (Weisbord *et al.* 1978; Roos *et al.* 1974), each of which have their own concept of what information is 'true' and 'valid'. What is relevant, valid information becomes a contested issue, prone to different interpretations more heavily influenced by organisational culture, internal politics and individual perceptions than any 'objective' rationales (Coyne, 1985a, 1985b).

3 *Healthcare organisations have lacked an information or IT culture.* The two issues described above have hindered investment in and utilisation of information systems in the English NHS. Many English healthcare organisations face a long learning curve in which to adapt a culture where information is used actively. Further, there has been under-investment in information systems in the NHS until the late 1980s (Kenny 1986), hence little tradition of using information systems at local operational level.

Local managers and information users consequently lack information skills and knowledge.

Healthcare organisations face specific problems in implementing information systems due to the very nature of health work which requires high professional input and autonomous professional decision making (Atkinson 1981; Freidson 1970; Kennedy 1981). Examples of the resulting problems for the role of information systems can be seen in the implementation of information systems in the NHS over the past 10 years. The author's own studies of the perceptions of resource management project managers and nurses (at the Health Services Management Unit, University of Manchester) during 1990–1 suggest that they perceive:

1 The biggest barrier to change was a lack of funds to implement the information systems into developing organisational structures properly.
2 Their biggest success was to involve clinicians in managerial processes.
3 The most important skill required to implement resource management was change management, which was ranked as more important than information skills or knowledge.
4 The respondents thought that resource management was not universally understood or known by their colleagues or staff.
5 A need for training staff about using information.

A similar study of medical records managers' perceptions of implementing Resource Management (RM) discovered that often medical records managers were not significantly involved in the implementation process, which adversely affected their motivation to change working practices (Aldridge and Walker 1991). These studies suggest that Resource Management, like most information systems projects, is a broad ranging organisational change which relies on involving all staff who will be affected by the change through good communication and process management skills. Training also can facilitate the progress of introducing what was perceived as a wide-ranging and sensitive change.

Contrary to much opinion, successful implementation of a computer based information system does not depend only on technical expertise. Because information systems and their accompanying technology critically affect the working of organisations and their staff, broader expertise is required to implement information systems with success. A purely technical approach may ignore the fact that information systems function within an organisational context (Galbraith 1977; Tichy 1978). (For instance, Resource Management systems were intended to provide management information on the use of finance.) Yet many information systems fail to meet the broader objectives of the organisations in which they are implemented. A recent report on NHS information systems applications by the National Audit Office (1990) noted a consistent failure 'to meet project objectives'. Those implementing these systems had lost from view the key objective of the organisation and thus of the rationale for the systems themselves.

Methodologies for implementing information systems

To overcome the problem of implementing information systems to comply with an organisational context several methodologies have been invented ('methodologies' in the informatic sense of the word; see Chapter 1). This section outlines and critically assesses three of the best-known.

Structured systems design

Because information systems inevitably involve technology much has been made of their technical requirements. Yet there has been a steady movement away from the traditional method of developing information systems over the past twenty years. Managers have become aware that a technical approach looking purely at the function of information in the organisation and ignoring the affects of information in the social or cultural contexts is dangerously narrow (Blackler and Brown 1986; Hirschheim 1985a). While a purely technical approach is effective in designing database structures, hardware or software requirements, there is little awareness of how an information system may be perceived by groups who traditionally do not identify with information systems, a good example being the medical profession. Any system designed without considering this will be incompatible with the organisational needs described above, hence unwanted and inefficient (Eason 1982); a false investment. Instead Blackler and Brown (1986) identified two distinct strands of system implementation:

1 task and technology
2 organisation and end user.

Socio-technical design

One approach which emerged as a growing awareness of the failure of 'rationalistic' methods of introducing information systems was the socio-technical approach to designing information systems. The SSADM method sees the need for integrating the technical features with the social (i.e. the culture and social networks) aspects of the change provoked by the information systems (see Figure 7.1). The logic of this approach is that organisations and the individuals which work in them are not purely logical 'systems', but rather have broader social needs and functions which need to be considered as well (Bostrom *et al.* 1977; Cherns 1987).

Nevertheless, criticisms can be made of the socio-technical design methodology. Chisholm and Zeigenfuss (1986) argued that the complex nature of

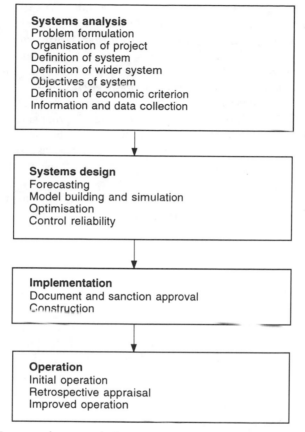

Systems analysis
Problem formulation
Organisation of project
Definition of system
Definition of wider system
Objectives of system
Definition of economic criterion
Information and data collection

Systems design
Forecasting
Model building and simulation
Optimisation
Control reliability

Implementation
Document and sanction approval
Construction

Operation
Initial operation
Retrospective appraisal
Improved operation

Figure 7.1   Structured systems design

healthcare organisations posed a dilemma for the socio-technical approach which attempts to bring together the technical and social systems into an integrated whole. In one case of implementing technical change they discovered 60 main tasks which had to be integrated into a technical option, leaving a large task for the change agents. Another criticism of a socio-technical approach in healthcare organisations is that their 'social' systems are just as complex, if not more so, than their technical systems. Passmore *et al.* (1986) discovered that the 'specialization and class structure of the health care environment posed unusual challenges to a Socio-Technical Systems application'. Healthcare organisations are 'characterized by the tendency towards diverse goals, diffuse authority, low task inter-dependence' (Weisbord 1976). This creates what Maslow (1972) termed 'low synergy organisations' where systems are dependent on each other for the organisation to work. Yet staff see themselves not as interdependent but as owing allegiance to their own particular department (Oaker and Brown 1986) or profession. There is great complexity in the number of social systems and how they interact. Another problem with using socio-technical methodologies design in hospitals is that healthcare organisations often have large professional groups who need to be actively involved in defining the terms of reference of any new information system, especially if the information it generates has managerial overtones (Passmore *et al.* 1986).

Several studies conclude that implementing change in healthcare organisations through traditional organisational development techniques (for example, Boss 1989) which focus on prescriptive methods (e.g. McDaniel *et al.* 1987) and mirror dominant managerial cultures, are essentially flawed (Weisbord 1976; Petee and Bastian 1986) because of the highly convoluted organisational structures, processes and cultures. What is required is a means of introducing information systems which concentrates on process and is neutral between the potentially conflicting cultures and sub-cultures, but allows full exploration of all issues which are relevant to managers and staff within the organisation.

Participative design

As a result of the recognition of the problems inherent in the process of socio-technical design the participative method of designing information systems grew more popular from the late 1970s. Like the socio-technical approach this method recommends balancing the social and the technical factors in an organisational change. It differs from the socio-technical approach in recommending that all members of the organisation be actively involved in designing and implementing the information system. There are several reasons for involving potential users of an information system in its design. It has been suggested that it is 'a good thing' in ethical principle to do so (Sashkin 1984), and an essential part of improving the working life of staff. There will be less resistance to change if individuals can influence this (Hirschheim 1985b; Mumford 1983a). Also the people who know how the system should fit into the organisational dynamics are often the users themselves (Mumford 1983b; Land and Hirschheim 1986). If the system is not implemented prescriptively it has a better chance of fitting into the context of the organisation which it will serve. Users often know their information requirements. The problem with health services is that there are likely to be many information requirements supporting a variety of tasks and individuals. Each of these demands for information is valid. Involving the users throughout system design and implementation reduces the danger of looking at information needs prescriptively (Klein and Hirschheim 1987; Mitroff and Mason 1983).

A well-known participative methodology was developed by Mumford (1983a). Figure 7.2 outlines it.

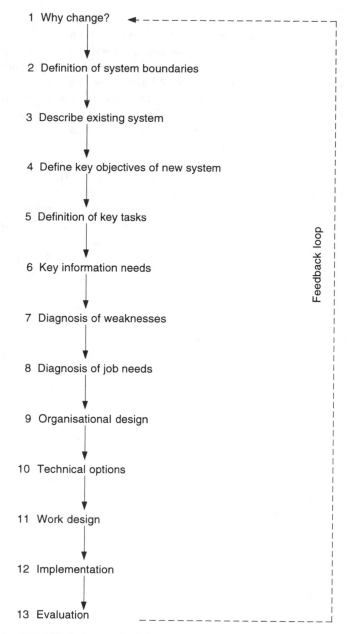

Figure 7.2   ETHICS design methodology

ETHICS (Effective Technical and Human Implementation of Computer Based work Systems) is a simple methodology comprising a series of defined procedures, as follows:

1 *Why change?* The first step in the ETHICS methodology asks a basic question which is often overlooked. Why instigate change? To change the way of doing things in an organisation, for example by developing an information system, requires effort, investment and patience. Often things can go wrong. So there should always be benefits emerging from change. The potential benefits of the change should be identified beforehand by those who are leading the process, and disseminated throughout the organisation so a strong vision and belief for change is held by all in the organisation.

2 *Define system boundaries.* The second step is to define the boundaries of the future system: What the system will be concerned with? Defining the system boundaries does not mean that the technical specifications are defined. Rather it concerns in broad terms what the outputs of the system, namely information, are intended to do and what part this information will have in the functioning of the organisation.

3 *Description of the existing system.* If a system is being developed it often replaces another system. There should be description of the previous system to ensure compatibility between systems and that the good aspects of the older system are built upon and developed in the new system. These may be technical hardware or software aspects but are more likely to be system procedures.

4 *Definition of key objectives.* The basic objectives of the system should be defined next, dictating the operational and managerial terms of reference for the system. For instance, will the system have the objective of providing financial information or personnel information? The objectives also dictate the terms of evaluation (see below, point 13).

5 *Definition of key tasks.* Definition of the key tasks of the system is essential. They should be defined at an early stage because they determine the technical requirements of the system. Ideally, the definition of key tasks should be formulated in the abstract so that the ideal requirements of the system are placed within the broader organisational and managerial needs. The key tasks are not constraints in any way.

6 *Key information needs.* The key information needs relate to those functions the system will provide information for within the organisation. The questions which need to be asked here are: what specific information do we want from the system; how do these fit into the objectives and tasks defined in stages 4 and 5?

7 *Diagnosis of potential weaknesses.* The potential weaknesses and constraints of the system should be anticipated now. When designing the system the things which the system cannot do need to be considered.

8 *Diagnosis of job satisfaction needs.* The development of an information system needs to take into account how individuals' working lives will change. There needs to be an investigation of what job satisfaction individuals require to use the system to its full potential. As

Mumford (1972) showed, if individuals are not satisfied in their work their performance suffers, reducing the effectiveness of any newly developed system.

9 *Organisational design.* The design of the organisational functions and procedures which are connected with the proposed system need to be clearly thought through, so as to incorporate the information system into the organisation's decision-making processes, to ensure maximum effectiveness of the information (Galbraith 1974). Tichy (1977) argued that any organisational design for healthcare organisations requires an integrated process which includes socio-technical aspects.

10 *Technical options.* The technical specifications of any newly developed system need to be looked at after the nine issues above have been determined and a clear strategy developed. The technical aspects are often the most flexible aspects of system design and implementation because clear specifications can be defined, developed and met. The constraints faced by technical specifications are also clearer than the managerial and human constraints, which emerge over time. Technical considerations are subordinate to the managerial and organisational considerations for any information system.

11 *Work design.* Work design is important. It ensures that the information system is compatible with the organisational structures and processes.

12 *Implementation.* Implementation of the information system needs to be carefully managed with specified deadlines and criteria for reaching them. In short, this is a typical project management exercise. However, one fundamentally different aspect within the participative style is that all individuals, irrespective of their status, should be able to contribute to the implementation strategy. The implementation strategy should include:
   (a) an assessment of the time requirements of the project
   (b) an assessment of resource implications of implementation
   (c) identification of who will be affected by it
   (d) what extra skills (if any) are needed to implement the system?
   (e) what are the constraints on the project?

13 Evaluation. Any system which has been implemented and developed should be thoroughly, properly and formally evaluated to ensure that:
   (a) it meets all the defined and desired objectives
   (b) lessons are learnt from implementing it
   (c) future system developments can build on the system implemented.

Implementing information systems participatively

The benefits of participative design methods for managing organisational change in healthcare organisations have been found in several studies (Aldridge *et al.* 1988; Stoelwinder and Clayton 1978; Weisbord and

Stoelwinder 1979). A study of implementing computer-based accountancy systems in a Swedish hospital found that clinicians were well intentioned towards the new systems if they had had a say in the formation of those systems (Coombes 1987). In a study of resource management systems implementation the authors (Aldridge and Walker 1991) also found that if clinicians were involved then they perceived benefits of the system as higher. If users of the intended systems were involved, awareness of information and its supporting technology was raised, helping bring a broader 'information culture' into the organisation. An evaluation of participative methods of implementing strategic decision support information systems (King and Rodriguez 1991) found no conclusive objections to the approach, and suggested that although the tangible benefits may appear small its other benefits are improved organisational communication and a more creative climate for change.

Nevertheless the idea of designing and implementing information systems participatively has its critics. Blackler and Brown (1986) argue that the ETHICS methodology is naive about organisational politics; powerful individuals or groups dominate the choice of those with less power. Margulies and Black's (1987) analysis of participation and the implementation of quality strategies found that most resistance to the method and the change it developed came from middle managers who thought their power threatened by other work groups. This may be especially liable to occur in healthcare organisations with powerful professional groups.

So participative methods of designing and implementing information systems have advantages and disadvantages. The biggest pay-off for such an approach would seem to be if a system is to be implemented in an organisation fraught with possible conflict and tension. The benefits of participation would also seem to be greater when the system is to be used by, and will affect, diverse groups such as professionals and managers. These are precisely the conditions prevalent in healthcare organisations. With the changes of the 1980s the English NHS has also become more polarised between clinical and managerial cultures who are forced to meet head on over information systems.

Assuming participation is a 'good thing', and may also be a successful way of introducing information systems into healthcare organisations, the conditions for a successful participative approach need to be considered. Mohrman and Ledford (1985) stated that effective participative approaches need three things:

1 The necessary knowledge and skills, and formal procedures to integrate participative methods fully into organisational decision. In healthcare organisations this means using facilitators who are competent and independent.

2 To be vertically and horizontally integrated into the organisation.

3 To be a regular part of the organisation, its culture and decision making processes.

Pettigrew *et al.* (1988) identified one of the key problems with managing change in the NHS as the inability to turn broad ranging strategies into meaningful organisational change. An informatics strategy for healthcare organisations at a local level should anticipate how change is to be managed. Key elements of the change process need to be considered when information systems are being implemented.

Many theorists have written on the benefits of change through incremental stages (Cummings and Held 1985; Hinnings and Greenwood 1988; Quinn 1980; Starbruck and Nystrom 1981) as organisations themselves tend to 'evolve' through the interactions of their members rather than be created suddenly (Silverman 1970; Weick 1979). When the manager faces uncertain and risky outcomes of change an incremental approach with the emphasis on experiment is possibly the best strategy, allowing the organisation time to adapt and develop in line with the newly installed information system. However the limited timescales which many contemporary managers operate under means that an approach which attempts to 'get it right' first time also has attractions; it can be beneficial in terms of cost if it succeeds.

An implementation strategy should also consider the problems of implementing what is a potentially radical organisational change. Information system implementation is no exception, as a complex change arousing many fears among people. One dilemma is of managing the present systems while attempting to manage the change process, especially difficult in healthcare organisations where 'everything seems so needy' and as a result resources are scarce.

Clarity of purpose is essential if the new information system is to be implemented successfully, so that individuals who will be affected can see what the future is and so that the reason for introducing the change is never forgotten during implementation. Both those in control of implementing the information system and those on the receiving end need to believe that the new system will improve their ability to meet the organisation's objectives. There need to be key operating principles for the change process and the system when it is implemented. All such operating principles should be clearly connected to the purpose of the system, flexible enough to allow creativity in defining the project but stringent enough to allow effective project management and deadlines to be within the resources allocated.

Environmental constraints should be made explicit. One is the resourcing of the information system to be implemented. Another, often overlooked, is the complexity of the environment to be modelled by the information system. This is particularly relevant to community resource management systems.

Being aware of the environmental constraints allows those managing the change process to plan the implementation programme more carefully. It is important to plan how the project will progress from stage to stage, with realistic deadlines for completing the project definition, system definition, decision on hardware requirements and the implementation processes. Resistance to change is inevitable but the participative approach outlined above is one possible way to reduce it. By integrating systems one can ensure that different information systems are technically compatible and that staff do not have to acquire a multiplicity of unique skills.

The above sections argue the need to understand the process of developing information systems within the local context of the organisation where the systems are to be implemented. Various methodologies for implementing information systems have been described, but what is needed in the NHS is a combination of all the methods; a locally based strategy which takes the views of relevant people into account and which recognises the need for 'bottom up' information flows (Abbott 1986) rather than imposed 'top down' strategies. This is increasingly so as the NHS moves towards localised purchasing and providing, with individual NHS organisations having increasing power to determine their own information needs. When information systems are being implemented in healthcare organisations managers should therefore remember that:

1 Technical, organisational and managerial issues need equal attention, for information systems affect, and are affected by, all three.
2 Information systems development can be implemented to greater effect through an evolutionary approach which evaluates and considers each stage of the change process on its merits. Then individuals who resist change can slowly become used to new technology and ways of working. Organisational culture and operating procedures can adapt slowly to new information and its technology. The advantages and disadvantages of specific elements of the systems and the information it produces can be assessed in more detail, over a longer period. Mistakes in the implementation or assumptions in the design can more easily be rectified and are not so expensive, and the initial investment of money, time and other resources will be less.
3 The amount and range of training and organisational development which new information systems require to utilise them fully should not be underestimated. A training and developmental strategy for the information system and the wider organisation should be planned.
4 Users' concerns and wishes should be carefully listened to, so as to gain maximum support throughout the organisation. One way of doing this is to avoid discussing the future role of the information system in too technical terms.

The benefits of information systems are not only financial but in how that information aids the function of the organisation as a whole. Information may often be expensive to develop and maintain, but it is a worthwhile investment if it helps the organisation reach its objectives more effectively.

Chapter 8

HEALTH RECORDS

Lorraine Nicholson and Heather Walker

From medical records to health records

The medical record is the most important tool for healthcare information storage, retrieval and analysis. It is the repository of all information concerning the patient's history and health, diseases, health risks, diagnoses, prognoses, tests and examinations, treatment and follow up. It is also a main source of information for health management; quality assurance, health statistics, service utilisation analysis among other activities. Informatics support of healthcare therefore centres on and begins with the medical record system.

Reasons for using an informatics approach to medical records keeping are, first, that the quality of the medical record is increased in terms of completeness, legibility and standardisation. Communication between healthcare providers contributing to the care of the patient is improved, making continuity of care easier. Appropriate care and follow-up are facilitated. There is easier retrieval of information, health records are more complete, and organisation of the health record, recall systems, appointment scheduling systems and repeat prescription systems become more logical. Medical audit becomes easier and more accurate. Clinical research is facilitated by improved data collection and automatic analysis. Lastly, the accuracy and timeliness of national health statistics improve.

The GP record system was introduced in 1948 and is the only birth to death record. It is created when a patient is first registered with a GP from the birth notification and follows the patient around the country as he or she moves practices. The record, known as the 'Lloyd George envelope', measures 17 cm by 12 cm, is buff coloured with red ink for males and blue for females and is still used today. It has remained this size as it is easy for the GP to carry on home visits. The record is provided by the FHSA. Any GP wishing to use another size must finance this change and return the records to the Lloyd George envelope when the patient changes GP or dies.

Hospital medical records originally developed as single-speciality based records created by the healthcare professional responsible for a patient's treatment. In many hospitals they remained as such until the Tunbridge Report (Ministry of Health 1965) attempted to standardise medical records and record-keeping across England and Wales. The report also defined documentation within the medical record. This led to the introduction of a number for commonly used documents (e.g. form HMR1 as the front sheet). Over the years there has been considerable discussion as to the content of the medical record, what documents must be retained, which may be destroyed and the filing order of documents. A4 paper became more standard as did hospital-wide rather than speciality-based records. Above all records were now divided into three different types: primary, secondary and transitory. Tunbridge advocated different retention periods for each of the three. This advice has since been updated by *Health Circular (89)20*, legal requirements, advice from the RCS and guidance notes issued in 1989 and 1994 (NHSTD 1994) (see below).

The steering group on Health Services Information chaired by Edith Körner was appointed by the Secretary of State for Health and Social Services in 1980. Six main Körner reports were published between 1982 and 1984. The first, on Hospital Facilities and Diagnostic Services (DHSS 1982), had the largest impact on medical records departments and their information collection systems. Körner identified a minimum data set and statutory times for the collection of information, with additional items of data which could be collected for local use. Since the NHS reforms these minimum data sets have since been modified to meet the data requirements outlined in *Working for Patients: Framework for Information Systems: The Next Steps* (Department of Health 1990c).

These developments have resulted in the following varieties of health record being commonly used in the UK (besides the GP record already mentioned).

The *Problem Orientated Medical Record* designed by Dr Lawrence Weed (Weed 1969) requires the doctor to approach all the patients' problems, treating them individually. It consists of four parts:

1 *The database*, containing the patient's presenting complaint as expressed by the patient, a history of the complaint, past medical history and results of any physical examinations.
2 *The problem list*, at the front of the medical record. Each problem is, numbered, dated and described as either active, inactive or resolved.

3 *The initial plan* of the patient's care, using the problem list. It can include diagnostics, therapeutic and patient education.
4 *Progress notes* detailing the treatment given and any further plans, by individual problem.

The first type of *patient-held record* was the ante-natal cooperation card held by the patient and taken to both the GP and hospital doctor. Some health authorities introduced the patient-held medical record for maternity cases because they thought it important that the record be available wherever the patient was admitted or delivered. Patient-held maternity records are now used throughout the UK. They allow patients to keep information which they may not wish disclosed to their spouse or other family members confidential by the use of a separate record retained by the hospital. This record will also contain information that an obstetrician or midwife regard as likely to mislead the patient or cause her anxiety. Some trusts are now allowing patients access to their nursing and medical records while in hospital or before a consultation. The problems appear not to be in allowing the patient to read the record but in preventing access to third parties. The District Health Authorities operating such a system have found that patients treat the records very responsibly with negligible loss being reported. The system is also thought to have improved the doctor–patient relationship and saved clerical and secretarial time by reducing communication between the hospital and the patient's GP. Medical records staff saved time by not having to pull notes for clinics and re-filing afterwards as nearly all patients do not have separate records retained by the hospital.

An experiment in portable medical records for homeless mentally ill people was conducted in Tower Hamlets in 1988–89. This study showed that having a patient held medical record for homeless people is feasible (Reuler and Balazs 1991). The utility of the record was proved as patients presented it to various healthcare providers who were able to obtain a certain amount of basic information and a contact for future care. These providers were also able to contribute to the record and provide information previously unavailable. The most common reasons for a patient failing to bring the record was that the patient had forgotten or it had been stolen. The study concluded that a patient-held record for chronically mentally ill people could be used safely.

Parent-held child records developed by the British Paediatric Association are now available to UK Health Authorities following similar schemes in other countries. The record is A5 sized with a plastic cover. It costs between £1 and £2 per record and funding for this is presently being sought from the Department of Health. The records contain details of a child's development, behaviour and illnesses. Parents as well as clinicians can add to the record. It is not intended to replace the GP's record but will be immediately available whenever a child has contact with the health service and will supplement the record held by the GP or hospital. It has the advantage of being available even when families move to another area and register with a new GP.

General practitioners in Exmouth have experimented with a patient-held 'Care Card', a smart card which has been used to record information of allergies, operations, medication and the advice given. The smart cards were carried by the patient and 'read' whenever the patient visited their GP, hospital, pharmacist or dentist. It was also possible for patients to read some information from their own cards although they were not entitled to the full information on it (Department of Health 1990d). Although some work has been completed on smart-cards and optical cards to be held by the patient, the amount of information contained on the card and that accessible to the patient is still limited. A single health record from birth to death is still not a reality.

Security and confidentiality of health records

Technological developments naturally raise questions about the security and confidentiality of health records, for which Medical Records Managers have a unique dual responsibility. Responsibility for the security of documentation lies with the hospital or HA (as agent for the Secretary of State for Health). Responsibility for the security and confidentiality of information contained within the record lies with the clinicians who compiled the record.

HC(89)20 sets out hospital and health authority responsibilities for retaining, preserving and destroying personal health records. It recommends that a designated officer be responsible for all matters relating to these matters. All systems for the selection and preservation of public records must comply with the *Public Records Acts* 1958–67, and all NHS records are public records for this purpose. Records dated 1660 and before must be retained permanently. Records which are 60 years old or more may only be destroyed after consultation and agreement with the creators, owners and users and after consultation with the local record office. Procedures for destroying medical records must take account of the *Act of Limitation* 1975; the *Congenital Disabilities Act* 1976; and the *Consumer Protection Act* 1987. Courts may require medical records to be available for longer than specified in these Acts and so the Department of Health has issued the following retention guidelines:

1 Obstetric records: for 25 years, or eight years after the patient dies.
2 Children's records: until the patient's 25th birthday, or eight years after the patient dies.
3 Mental illness records: for 20 years, or eight years after the patient dies.
4 Other medical records: for eight years.

HC(89)20 recommends establishing a Committee with representation from all interested parties including clinicians to oversee all matters relating to the preservation, retention and destruction of medical records.

The *Data Protection Act* 1984 ratifies the Council of Europe *Data Protection Convention*. It also gives all citizens, employees and consumers a right of access to their personal data and safeguards the privacy of that data. Information terms are in special senses within the Act, and they include:

1 *Data* are defined as information recorded in a form in which it can be processed by equipment operating automatically in response to instructions given for that purpose.
2 *Personal data* are data relating to a living individual who can be identified from the information, including any expression of opinion or fact about that individual. The users' intentions towards the individual are not included.
3 A *data subject* is the living individual to whom the data relates. Corporate bodies, partnerships, etc. cannot be data subjects as the Act refers to 'individuals' and not 'persons'.
4 A *data user* is a person who processes or intends to process the data of a data subject.
5 *Computer bureaux* are organisations or individuals who process or provide back up facilities on personal data for data users on their equipment.
6 *Processing* is defined as amending, augmenting, deleting or re-arranging, or extracting information by means of reference to the data subject.
7 *Data classes* are the classification that data will be classified under. The data class will be related to the purpose chosen.
8 The *source* means 'the source from which it is intended to obtain the data'.

Figure 8.1 shows the bodies referred to in the Data Protection Act.

The *Data Protection Act* applies 'to the use of automatically processed information relating to living individuals and the provision of services in respect of such information'. All persons who are responsible for such data must be registered with the Data Protection Registrar. From 11 May 1986 it became illegal to hold and use personal computer-based data that has not been registered and approved by the Data Protection Registrar. Registration packs are available from all Post Offices. The Data Protection Register is available at all main libraries.

Anyone processing personal data automatically is legally required to register as a data user under the Act. A form which identifies the organisation and the purposes, uses, disclosures and sources of the data is completed and forwarded to the Data Protection Register with the appropriate fee. The Registrar may accept or reject the application. Successful applicants receive confirmation of acceptance and a copy of the details that have been entered in the Register, which is open to public inspection. The continued use of personal data on automated equipment following a rejected application (or in the case of failure to register) is an offence and the user could face prosecution. Domestic data users, unincorporated bodies and computer

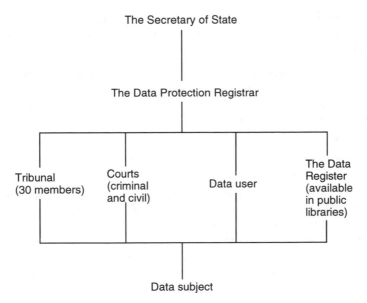

Figure 8.1 Bodies referred to in the Data Protection Act

bureaux (who are required only to register their name and address) may be exempt from registration.

Data users must adhere to the following principles of the Act:

1 The personal data must be obtained and processed fairly and lawfully.
2 The personal data must be held for specific purposes only.
3 The personal data must be compatible with the stated purposes and uses identified and not used or disclosed in any other manner.
4 The personal data must be adequate, relevant and not excessive.
5 The personal data must be accurate and kept up to date.
6 The personal data may not be held for longer than necessary.
7 Subject access must be effected without undue delay or expense.
8 Appropriate security measures must be taken against unauthorised disclosure, alteration, destruction, access and accidental loss of the personal data.

Data users who do not register computerised personal data applications (where living individuals can be identified from the data) are contravening the Data Protection Act and could face prosecution.

The Act gives data subjects the following rights:

1 To be informed by any data user whether personal data is held about them.
2 To be supplied with a copy of that data within 40 days of making a written request.
3 To have such data corrected or erased where appropriate.

A maximum of 40 days is allowed for this information to be made available to data subjects and a maximum fee of £10 is payable. The following procedure should be followed:

1 The data subject makes a written request to the data user and they may be required to provide evidence of identity.
2 The request must quote the Register entry number (obtainable from public libraries where the Register is available) and other information which the data user needs to identify the appropriate data.

A data subject will be denied access to information which can not be separated from data on another data subject, unless permission has been given. Data users have a statutory obligation to provide an explanation of unintelligible data held in coded form. Data subjects have the right of appeal to the Registrar or to the Courts in the event of any problems. In special circumstances a data subject may have the right of compensation for loss or destruction, unauthorised disclosure and inaccuracies. There is a limited right to have erroneous data rectified or erased. These rights are enforced through the Courts.

The Access to Personal Files Act 1987 gives individuals the right to see information held on them by Social Services Departments, Educational Authorities and Local Authorities. Under the Access to Medical Reports Act 1988 individuals have the right to see a doctor's report about them which has been compiled for an insurance company or an employer within 21 days of the report being compiled. They are also entitled to have incorrect information amended or deleted.

The Access to Health Records Act (1990f) gives patients a right to see information recorded in manually held medical or health records after 1 November 1990. The Act describes itself as:

> an Act to establish a right of access to Health Records, by individuals to whom they relate and other persons to provide for the correction of inaccurate health records and for the avoidance of certain contractual obligations; and for connected purposes.

The term 'health records' includes records held in NHS institutions, prisons, the armed forces, general practice, private treatment records and employment health records. Nothing in the Act prohibits voluntary informal arrangements to allow patients to see their records at the discretion of the health professional who is principally responsible for their clinical care but there must be no disclosure of information which might cause serious harm or which would identify any third parties. The Act is extensive. The Department of Health publishes Guidelines (Department of Health 1990g) for administration of the Access to Health Records Act 1990, which are available from HMSO.

The 1990 Act defines a health record as any information relating to the physical or mental health of an individual who can be identified from that information and which has been made by or on behalf of, a healthcare professional in connection with the care of that individual. The 'holder' of the health record is defined as the patient's GP (or if the patient does not have a GP, the FHSA or health board for the patient's most recently listed GP); or the health service body by which (or on whose behalf) the record is held; or, in any other case, as the health professional by whom (or on whose behalf) the record is held. The 'patient' is defined as the individual, in connection with whose care the record has been made. The Act defines a 'health professional' as any:

1 Registered medical practitioner.
2 Registered dentist.
3 Registered optician.
4 Registered pharmaceutical chemist.
5 Registered nurse, midwife or health visitor.
6 Registered chiropodist, dietician, occupational therapist, orthoptist or physiotherapist.
7 Clinical psychologist, child psychotherapist or speech therapist.
8 Art or music therapist employed by the health service.
9 Scientist employed by the health service as a head of department.

It gives a right of access to a patient's health record to:

1 The patient.
2 A person authorised in writing to apply on behalf of the patient.
3 The person having parental responsibility for a child patient (in England and Wales); or the parent or guardian where the patient is a pupil (in Scotland).
4 Any person appointed by the court to manage the affairs of a patient deemed to be incapable.
5 Where a patient has died, the patient's personal representative or any other person having a claim arising from the death.

For its purposes, the Act divides health information into two categories. 'Recent information' is that which has been recorded in the 40 days prior to the date of application for access to the record. The other category is of information recorded more than 40 days prior to the application but after 1 November 1991.

An application to inspect a health record or part of it must be made in writing. The health professional must be satisfied as to the identity and credentials of the applicant and where necessary must seek further information to establish or confirm the identity within 14 days of receiving the request. The statutory time limit for providing access commences from the date that the application has been accepted as valid and the fee, where appropriate, has been received. For recent notes (made within the 40 days immediately preceding the date of application) the record holder must allow access within 21 days. For notes relating to patients whose treatment has been completed and whose records have not been updated the record holder has 40 days in which to allow access. A fee may be charged for access to notes made more than 40 days prior to the application but after 1 November 1991, in line with fees allowed under the Data Protection Act (£10 in 1994). Additional charges may also be made to cover the costs of photocopying. No fees may be charged for access to notes made in the 40 days immediately prior to the date of application although charges for photocopying may be made. If a record contains terminology which is not understood by the patient an explanation of this terminology must be provided. The Act designates the General Practitioner as the holder of (GP) records, making access to GP records more straightforward than to other health records. Where a patient seeks access to their record and has no current GP the application should be made direct to the FHSA.

Access may be wholly denied to the following categories of applicant when the holder of the record is not satisfied that the patient is capable of understanding the nature of the application:

1 The patient.
2 A person authorised in writing to make application on behalf of the patient.
3 A child patient (in England and Wales); or a pupil patient (in Scotland). Here access may be denied if the holder is not satisfied that the patient has consented to the making of the application; or is not satisfied that the patient is capable of understanding the nature of the application; or is not satisfied that to grant access would be in the patient's best interests.

The Act provides for patients to request that access is not given after their death to their personal representative or to any person having a claim arising from the patient's death. This provision is not strictly enforceable as a patient ceases to have a legal personality after death. Where an application is on behalf of a child in England or Wales (or pupil, in Scotland), or where a patient is incapable of managing his own affairs, or has died, access to that part of information provided by the patient in the expectation that it would not be disclosed to the applicant may be refused. Access may also be refused, to information obtained as a result of examination or investigation, to which the patient consented in the expectation that the information would not be disclosed. Where a patient has died, access may not be given to any part of the record which, in the opinion of the holder, is not relevant to any claim which may arise out of the patient's death.

In certain circumstances access to the record may be denied in part. This may happen when the holder of the record believes that disclosure of that part may cause serious physical or mental harm to the patient or another individual, or where the information has been provided by a third party who could be identified from it. Access may also be denied where the record was compiled before the Act came into force (i.e. 1 November 1991), although access could be granted to records made before that date in order to make sense of subsequent records.

The health records service

The main responsibility of a health records or medical records department is to provide a record for every patient contact. The most difficult task of any health records department is tracing records through the system. Tracer systems have been greatly strengthened by the introduction of Patient Administration System (PAS) computerised tracking systems. The use of bar codes to aid the tracking of notes, and of additional PAS terminals, have enabled casenotes to be traced around hospital sites more easily and created some staff savings. For tracing and updating records maintaining unique patient identifiers is of paramount importance. Despite the Tunbridge Report there was no move towards a common NHS numbering or filing system, not even one using patients' NHS numbers, until the NHS new number project. This project is intended to provide a new NHS number by April 1995. The Administrative Register Project also aims to replace the numerous overlapping computer lists with a single comprehensive database. At first the Register will contain only information from the FHSA patient registers, with the aim of linking the register to hospital patient administration systems and child health registers. Each entry will contain an individual's name, date of birth, sex, address, NHS number and other details such as GP but will not contain patients' clinical details.

With the introduction of Resource Management (RMI) and the move towards the clinical directorate structure in some trusts, the medical records department has become decentralised and is no longer seen as a service department; the records library is all that remains of the central service. Benson (1991; p. 23) argues that:

> decentralisation of the patient administration functions is an opportunity still to be grasped. However, those responsible sometimes fail to realise that it is not only the department that they dismantle but the building block for the integrated hospital information systems. The move from any central service to a decentralised service has many implications, not all instantly recognisable.

A study in 1991 attempted to elicit project managers', project nurses' and other participants' perceptions of what impact the resource management initiative has had on medical records services (Aldridge and Walker 1991). The questionnaire also covered decentralisation of medical records departments and the debate about clinical coding. The results showed that despite the intentions of the RMI, medical records function coding were still heavily centralised. Medical records managers viewed Resource Management positively, as a way of facilitating the management process to promote better patient care. The results also indicated that common factors behind successful Resource Management were training managers and staff (see Chapter 10), developing change through participative methods (see Chapter 7) and early, effective communication on what Resource Management is and how it affects medical records. This suggests that those leading Resource Management activities need to recognise the role and importance of medical records in Resource Management information systems. It also suggests that they need to involve medical records managers, especially in linking medical records to case mix systems (see Chapter 5) and in anticipating the effect of Resource Management on departmental structures and roles. Medical records managers who wish to retain the coding function need to develop it in partnership with the clinicians (see Chapter 9).

Technical developments in health records

Informatics support for medical records comes in many forms. Some examples of current applications include micro-computers storing basic identification data about patients and providing a diagnostic index. Mini and mainframe applications store a complete medical record for each patient, including clinical text. Two technological developments are particularly promising.

Smart cards are credit-card sized pieces of plastic with a single microprocessor embedded in the plastic. The microprocessor stores not only the patient's health record but allows the card itself to control who looks at the record. The first use of such cards as health records was pioneered by Bull in 1985. In Blois (between Paris and Tours) smart cards were issued to everyone aged over 65, all babies and expectant mothers. Following this trial smart cards are being used by health services in Austria, Belgium, Canada, Italy, Spain and the USA. The NHS Care Card experiment develops this idea.

In 1989 Bull, Abies and the Department of Health started the first UK trial of smart card technology. A three-year project in Exmouth was to assess the benefits of a smart card system which transferred medical summaries and prescriptions electronically between GPs, pharmacists, dentists, hospital staff and clinicians. Eight thousand and five hundred patients from two general practices, and almost every diabetic in Exmouth, were issued with cards which could be read at all eight pharmacies in the town, one dental practice, the casualty department of Exmouth Hospital and Exeter District General Hospital. Read codes (see Chapter 9) were used to ensure information accuracy, consistency and completeness. The advantages of the system were portability of the card, instant access by the hospitals to information on drug regimes, GP clinical information and next of kin information. The cards improved the flow of accurate, timely information and enhanced the continuity of care. Common access to information was provided while maintaining total security of the information on the card. Patients' attitudes to the smart cards were reported as 'overwhelmingly positive'.

Optical cards are plastic cards that are the size of credit cards that can write and read two megabytes of data. They are portable, have a large data capacity and are relatively inexpensive. Data are recorded onto optical cards as digital signals and the cards can be connected to different types of system equipment and networks to provide a flexible, efficient configuration. Data can be added to the card but not erased.

Smart cards and optical cards show how a patient-held records system can enhance the continuity of patient care. They will offer significant opportunities as European boundaries open up after 1992.

Optical imaging systems are also being developed. Optical discs are a highly efficient storage medium which can hold any digitised image received via an optical scanner or facsimile machine. An optical disc is a 'write once, read many' (WORM) device. A single 30 cm disc can store up to 40,000 A4 sized images using compressed data for higher density storage. These disks are very reliable and durable. They are used within an integrated image processing system which combines a number of technologies. Briefly, these include input devices to capture document images; storage systems to maintain the image files; and data bases to provide indexing systems for locating individual images to facilitate retrieval. Indexing can be done on a keyboard or by using Intelligent Optical Character Recognition (IOCR). Image-capable workstations for viewing documents are part of the retrieval process, as are laser printers to produce hard copies and communication systems to send and print the images.

Clinical workstations and Electronic Patient Records (EPRs) are being developed through several large national projects as part of the national IM&T strategy (see Chapter 2). The Integrated Clinical Workstation (ICWS) is a short term, practical step but also part of a coherent approach towards introducing the electronic patient record. For the ICWS project to succeed it must be clinically driven and give advantage to clinicians at the point of delivery of care. Ethical and legal issues and concerns about data security and confidentiality must also be addressed as this is critical to generating confidence in clinical computer systems. Equally critical are the development of standards for data storage, the communication of images, a minimum data set and a core specification (which must also be agreed with the clinicians). The resulting systems must be flexible enough to cope quickly with change and able to support communications across primary, community and acute care. A number of technical archiving problems will also have to be resolved.

If successful, the ICWS project offers a number of benefits. The most important is to facilitate and improve clinical practice, improving patient care. For this, ICWS data must be person-based, use each patient's new NHS number as its unique patient identifiers), and include National Administrative Register data. Such a system would enable healthcare practitioners to adopt Read terms (see pp. 138–9) in their routine clinical practice and record data in whatever manner they consider optimal. It will help members of different professions work as one clinical team. Besides supporting the contracting function, it would provide the functional core, and basic data, for an electronic patient record.

Three main models for electronic patient record are emerging. *Finance based EPRs* are a short version of a comprehensive patient record. Their information core is financial, for billing and contracting purposes. *Provider-based EPRs* allow each provider unit to develop its own EPR content, structure and equipment. Each provider develops its EPR separately, unlinked to other providers. *Provider-linked EPRs* allow the development of compatible systems within each provider unit. They require each provider to be a curator of data; to store data securely, monitor data protection requirements, etc. Networking allows access by each healthcare professional discipline. This model requires compatible computer systems, compatible software, a common data structure and networking. Provider-linked EPRs seems to be the model that the NHS is most likely to adopt eventually.

The clinical workstation is a step along the way. Many of the components for the development of the clinical workstation are in place or being established. These include the NHS Data Dictionary, the Clinical Terms Project, new Read codes (see Chapter 9) and new NHS patient numbers.

NHS Data Dictionary, inaugurated in July 1993 and based on the Minimum Data Set Model Version 3.0. These data standards will apply to the whole NHS. The National Administrative Register will hold a common administrative data set across the whole NHS. The Clinical Terms Project involves doctors, nurses and paramedical professions, organised in 43 specialist groups. It has been reviewing lists of clinical terms with the intention of producing integrated thesaurus of clinical terms by April 1994. It will cross-reference these to ICD 10 and OPCS 4 (to ensure Read codes continue to support collection of data for central returns). The new terms will be published with a new version of the Read Codes (version 3; see Chapter 9). NHSME intend that replacement NHS patient numbers in their new format will be released in July 1995, with roll out to electronic GP information systems completed by December 1995, and to manual GP systems by April 1996.

New information technology is likely to have a major impact on medical record systems. Large data bases are a case in point. A lot of work is currently being done to provide population health registers and this may result in a common database for all hospitals, clinics and surgeries in a district. All health workers could have access to the medical records of a patient and record linkage could be achieved using the NHS number. This is technically possible but it poses many ethical issues regarding security and confidentiality.

Chapter 9

CLASSIFICATION AND CODING

Heather Walker

Classification, nomenclatures and coding

The statistical study of disease began for all practical purposes with the work of John Graunt on the London *Bills Of Mortality* in the early part of the eighteenth Century. Graunt undertook his study in an attempt to discover the number of babies dying before the age of six years. There were no records of age at death and so to establish their number he added all the deaths classified as thrush, convulsions, rickets, worms, abortives, chrysomes, infants liver-grown and overlaid half the deaths classified as smallpox, swine pox, measles and worms without convulsions. Despite the crudity of his methods he estimated that the mortality rate was 36 per cent before the age of six years and from later evidence this appears to have been a good estimate. Subsequently Francois Bossier de Lacroix (1706–77), better known as Sauvages, made a systematic classification, published as the treatise *Nosologia Methodica* (WHO 1977). A contemporary of his, Lillaeus (1708–78), also published a classificatory treatise entitled *Genera Morborum* (WHO 1977). By the late eighteenth century the classification of diseases had become one of the main methods of developing proto-scientific theories in western medicine (Foucault 1973).

By the early nineteenth Century the most widely used classification was one developed by William Cullen (1710–90) of Edinburgh, published as *Synopsis Nosologiae Methodicae* (Cullen 1769). The new General Registrar Office of England and Wales recruited William Farr as its first Medical Statistician in 1837. He worked to secure better and internationally uniform classifications, using Cullen's classification in his own work. His account of the aims of a statistical classification of disease still holds good:

> any classification that brings together in groups diseases that have considerable affinity, or that are liable to be confounded with each other, is likely to facilitate the deduction of general principles ... Several classifications may, therefore, be used with advantage; and the physician, the pathologist, or the jurist each from his own point of view, may legitimately classify the diseases and the causes of death in the way that he thinks best adapted to facilitate his inquiries, and to yield general results. (Farr (1856), appendix: 75–6)

In 1835, Farr and Marc d'Esprine of Geneva were charged with preparing a uniform nomenclature of causes of death in every country. By 1855 they had produced two separate lists based on different principles. A compound list was produced (and revised in 1864, 1874, 1880 and 1886); a direct ancestor of today's *International Classification of Diseases and Causes of Death* (WHO 1977). In 1891, the International Statistical Institute requested Jacques Bertillon to prepare a classification of causes of death. The current *International Statistical Classification of Diseases and Causes of Death* (WHO 1977) is a revision – the ninth – of Bertillon's original work of 1893. Published in 1975, it came into international use in 1979, being implemented in England and Wales during that year and in Scotland during 1980.

Some lists of diseases and operations are known as 'classifications', others as 'nomenclatures'. The differences between them were defined in 1965 by an expert group on Medical Terminology and Lexicography convened by the International Organisation for Medical Services. This group defined a classification as:

> a list of all the concepts belonging to a well defined group (e.g. of diagnoses, etc.) compiled in accordance with criteria enabling them to be arranged systematically, and permitting the establishment of a hierarchy based on the natural or logical relationship between them. A classification should not be confused with a nomenclature. Whereas the latter is simply a list of names, a classification is an attempt to establish a logical hierarchy between the concepts themselves. The name of a concept may change without affecting the place of the concept in the classification.

The differences were further emphasised by the definition of a nomenclature as:

> a systematic list, in one or several languages, of all or as many names as possible of members of a clearly defined conceptual or linguistic family, usually without accompanying definitions. Thus the names of all plants

constitute a botanical nomenclature and so with animals, tumours, diseases, etc.

So, in brief, a nomenclature of disease or surgical operations is a list of names, while a classification is a logical hierarchy of concepts. The distinction between the terms has become blurred as there is an obvious advantage in listing a nomenclature in a logical order. Classification serves as the basis for both coding and grouping systems in automated healthcare information systems, as the next two sections explain.

The main current classification and coding systems

For verbal data to be recorded and communicated electronically they have to be put into information systems in coded form. If the data are to be collatable and comparable, completely standard codes must be used throughout each information system, and by all information systems which share the data. Many clinical coding systems have been devised for this purpose, based on classification systems constructed on the principles outlined in the previous section. Some are speciality specific, others aim to be comprehensive. Some classify diseases, others the interventions used. This chapter introduces the classification and coding systems most commonly used in the UK. Outside the UK other systems are sometimes used: *Adaptation Hospitaliere des Maladies et des Operations* (HCIMO) in Belgium and Russia; NLSO in the Nordic countries; CDAM and THESAM in France; INAMI in Belgium; the *Vereinigung Schweizerischer Krankenhauser* system (VESKA) in Switzerland; International Classification of Clinical Services (ICCS) and Systematized Nomenclature of Medicine (SNOMED) in the USA. Work is under way to produce a pan-European system, at least for surgical procedures (Roger-France 1993).

The *International Statistical Classification of Diseases and Causes of Death* (ICD) is a statistical classification system promoted by the World Health Organisation so that experiences in different countries can be recorded in a similar way and compared. The first of its two volumes is the tabular list of diseases, the second an alphabetic index. The ninth revision of ICD (ICD9) contains the innovation of a dual classification of certain diagnostic statements. These descriptions contain elements of information about the generalised disease process in addition to the local manifestation or complication, showing both cause and effect of diseases. ICD9 also contains supplementary classifications known as 'E codes', 'V codes' and 'M codes'. E codes record external factors (e.g. injury, poisoning) associated with the diseases classified. V codes code other factors which influence health status and contact with health services. M codes classify malignant neoplasms by histological type and behavioural characteristics.

ICD9 was the first revision of ICD to include a classification of procedures in medicine. Although some countries, notably the USA, had for some time been including classifications of surgical procedures in their national adaptations of ICD9, international accord in this area had never been achieved and the classification of procedures had never been included in the main classification itself.

The WHO's *ICD9 International Classification of Procedures in Medicine* (ICPM) (WHO 1977) is a procedure code book intended to be applicable to both outpatients and inpatients. It includes all types of procedures for statistical, administrative, clinical or research purposes, encompassing exploratory, radiological, surgical and other diagnostic, prophylactic or therapeutic procedures. ICPM is organised into nine chapters covering:

1 procedures for medical diagnosis
2 laboratory procedures
3 radiology and certain other applications of physics in medicine
4 preventive procedures
5 surgical operations
6 and 7 drugs, medicaments and biological agents
8 other therapeutic procedures
9 ancilliary procedures.

The *International Classification of Diseases, 9th Revision, Clinical Modification* (ICD–9-CM) is based on the official version of ICD9 and also draws heavily on ICPM (USNCPHA 1986). The modification is to extend the classification to include morbidity data, for example on disease staging, and to extend ICD9 into a grouping system (Roger-France 1993; see the next section). To describe the clinical state of the patient ICD–9-CM codes must be more precise than the ICD9 codes sufficient for statistical groupings and trend analysis. The modified classification is used for indexing medical records, medical care review, and ambulatory and other medical care programmes besides basic health statistics. The decision to create a clinical modification was based not only on the need for increased specificity but also on several other facets of ICD–9, notably on complications of pregnancy, childbirth and the puerperium, where it was previously impossible to tell if a patient had delivered or if certain complications occurred before, during or after delivery. Of equal concern was the dual classification scheme in ICD9 which provided an alternative code for classifying some conditions according to aetiology or manifestation depending on the interest of the user (USNCPHA 1986).

ICD9-CM is published in three volumes. Volume 1 contains the tabular list of diseases and four appendices (a morphology of neoplasms; a glossary of mental disorders; a classification of drugs by American Hospital Formulary Service List number and their ICD9-CM equivalents; and a classification of industrial accidents according to agency). Volume 2 is the alphabetical index and Volume 3 contains both the tabular list and the alphabetical index of procedures. The publication has been expanded to include health related conditions and to provide greater specificity at the fifth digit level of detail.

The tenth revision of the *International Classification of Diseases* (ICD10) (WHO 1992) is due to be introduced from 1995. Discussions on the revision have continued since 1983. In 1984 and 1986 WHO circulated drafts to member states, speciality groups and individual experts. The British response was coordinated by OPCS. ICD10 will contain some fundamental departures. It will for the first time be published in three volumes, Volume 1 being the tabular list, Volume 2 coding and other instructions for its use, and Volume 3 an alphabetical index. Chapters will now take an alpha-numeric format. The number of chapters increases from 17 to 21 with the previous supplementary chapters (relating to external causes and factors influencing health status) being included in the numbered sequence. These changes increase ICD10's capacity to almost double that of ICD9. The full title of the classification has also been changed, reflecting the inclusion of the supplementary chapters in this revision, to the *International Statistical Classification of Diseases and Related Health Problems* but will fortunately retain the abbreviation 'ICD'.

An early British classification system was devised by the Medical Research Council. Using a simple system of three digit codes suitable for processing by the punch card equipment available at the time it identified 443 categories of operation. The 1956 version contained 674 categories together with the radiotherapeutic and anaesthetic supplements. It was the first version to be used for the Hospital Inpatient Enquiry (HIPE). However, this application revealed some not previously apparent inadequacies which led to a further revision in 1962 (published in 1969), although RHAs used a draft version from 1967 for the coding of Hospital Activity Analysis records. The revised version again increased the categories available, this time to 731, but the major change was to introduce an optional fourth digit extension in almost half the categories. A further revision in 1975 was prompted partly by a desire to ensure some compatibility with the anticipated WHO *International Classification of Procedures in Medicine* and therefore included considerable expansion at the fourth digit categories despite the UK central government requirement remaining at the three-digit level.

The Office of Population Censuses and Surveys was formed in 1970 by amalgamating the General Register Office and the Government Social Survey. The General Register Office had previously been responsible for registering births, deaths and marriages, for undertaking censuses and for providing a range of medical and population statistics. The division works closely with the World Health Organisation and is concerned with the coding and analysis of causes of death and illness. Its other areas of work include cancer registration, notification of infectious diseases, abortion statistics and the national morbidity study carried out on behalf of the Department of

Health. The Office of Population Censuses and Surveys produce a *Classification of Surgical Operations* (OPCS4) whose present (fourth) revision appeared in 1987 (OPCS 1987). It draws on a system of classifying surgical operations dating back to 1944.

The latest development was instigated by the Steering Group on Health Services Information (DHSS 1982) chaired by Edith Körner who reported that 'the 1975 revision was by then several years out of date due to the continuous movement towards new operative techniques' (DHSS 1982). Körner therefore recommended that OPCS should urgently provide operation codes that reflected current practice. Three classification systems already in use elsewhere were considered for adoption in Britain but as all three were deficient in some areas, particularly vascular and cardiac surgery, and were themselves in need of revision, it was agreed to revise the existing OPCS classification.

The *Read Clinical Classification* (NHSME 1993d) is a coded nomenclature of medical terms for use by clinicians, developed by James Read, a Loughborough GP. It consists of alphanumeric codes with one to five character levels and 58 possible branches at each level giving a theoretical maximum of 656 356 768 available 'Read codes'. The classification is cross referenced to all of the widely used standard classifications (ICD9, ICD–9-CM, OPCS4, British National Formulary) and will be mapped to ICD10. The classification codes not only diseases but also patient history and symptoms, examination findings and signs, diagnostic procedures, preventive, operative, therapeutic and administrative procedures, drugs and appliances and occupations and social information. The aim is to use terms that clinicians know and understand, to enable them to classify in as much detail as possible with a unique code. Read codes also allow the description of particular events in the order in which they happen, from initial presentation with signs and symptoms through to investigations, final diagnosis and treatment.

Version 2 of the file structure for Read codes was designed to improve the usability of the codes for clinical purposes. A 'term code' has been developed that records the actual term used by the clinician. The user's term is then used for retrieval and reporting instead of the system's preferred default term (so that, for instance, the system uses 'heart attack' rather than 'acute myocardial infarction' when reporting back to its user). This has been achieved by extending the 'term keys' used for finding terms from four to 10 characters in length, allowing faster, more efficient scrutiny of terms when drawing up a picking list. Version 3 contains a new file structure, prompted by the needs for forward and backward compatibility with ICD9 and ICD10; to accommodate the much greater detail in clinical information arising from Clinical Terms Project; and for a more elegant on-screen display of terms. Existing Read code formats and associated text descriptions remain unchanged and all current five-byte Read codes will be carried through to Version 3.

Read codes' advantages were first recognised in 1988 by the Joint Computing Group of the Royal College of General Practitioners and by the General Medical Services Committee. They were mainly concerned with classification in primary care and recommended the adoption of the Read Clinical Classification as the standard classification of general practice data in the United Kingdom. This group went on to promote the adoption of the Read codes universally by the NHS which led to the acquisition of the codes by the Department of Health in 1990. Licensing and supporting the use of Read codes is the responsibility of Computer Aided Medical Systems Limited who provide technical support and training courses for system suppliers. The next step is for the NHS Centre for Coding and Classification to continue to develop the Read codes through its work with the medical and paramedical colleges and through the speciality groups.

Diagnosis related groups and other grouping systems

Various grouping systems have become available, derived in part from the coding systems described in preceding sections. However grouping systems differ from classification systems in two ways. Existing grouping systems group patients who have already been allocated a clinical classification system code (say an ICD9 or a Read code); and group them according to further, non-clinical criteria (usually financial criteria). Of these grouping systems, Diagnostic Related Groups are the most widely known both in the United Kingdom (see Bardsley *et al.* 1987) and the European Union (see Roger-France *et al.* 1989). United States grouping systems include Current Physicians' Terminology (CPT3), Patient Management Categories (PMCs) and attempts to extend ICD–9-CM into a grouping system by adding disease staging or procedure codes to ICD9.

Diagnosis related groups (DRGs) are a patient grouping scheme which relates patients' clinical types to the costs incurred, for patients discharged from acute hospitals. DRGs were developed in the late 1960s at Yale University and implemented initially in New Jersey in the late 1970s as the basis for a prospective payment system. In 1984 they were adopted by US Medicare for their Prospective Payment System for hospitals.

The purpose of the DRG system is to enable healthcare purchasers to standardise for the effects of different case mixes when comparing the costs of using different hospitals. DRGs can be used to show the proportions of simple or complicated, cheap or costly cases admitted and how these frequencies vary for different hospitals, specialities or consultants. One derives DRGs by grouping together those clinical classifications whose treatment costs per patient are similar. (This is why DRGs are sometimes described as 'iso-resource' groups; the costings are normally in money but there have been experiments with costing in terms of healthworker time (Petit

1989)). Next for each group, the ratio of its per-patient treatment cost to the mean cost of treating a patient (averaged over all clinical categories) is calculated. The resulting 'DRG weights' can then be used to analyse and compare the total bills presented to a healthcare purchaser by each provider (for further explanation see Bardsley *et al.* 1987; ProPAC 1991; Sheaff and Peel 1993). A DRG analysis also shows how cases were managed in terms of length of stay, cost and other inputs. Resource needs can then be calculated for future service plans and used to estimate costs, set and monitor budgets both at purchaser and at provider levels (see also Chapters 2, 3 and 12). In practice DRG analyses incidentally provide an audit of complete or usable patient records.

DRGs are based on the fact that while patients are unique they also have demographic, diagnostic and therapeutic attributes in common. To be effectively usable DRGs need to be medically coherent, genuinely iso-resource, derived from routinely available data and to contain a manageable number of categories. In the DRG system all possible principal diagnoses are divided into 23 mutually exclusive principal diagnosis areas referred to as major diagnostic categories. The majority of the major diagnostic categories are then divided into medical or surgical groups. Surgical categories are defined by the precise surgical procedure performed. Medical categories defined by the principal diagnosis for which the patient was admitted. The categories are then defined into the 470 DRGs. Then each class of patient is evaluated to determine if complications or co-morbidities, age or discharge status would consistently affect the consumption of hospital resources. (A complication or co-morbidity is defined as a condition that increases the length of stay by at least one day in 75 per cent of patients.) The patient's age is also in some cases a factor influencing their assignment to a DRG. A final determinant in some cases is the discharge status, with alternative DRGs being formed for burn patients, newborns, patients transferred to another acute care facility, patients with alcoholism or drug abuse, patients who left against medical advice, and for acute myocardial infarction patients and newborns who died.

Given their connection with cost control it is not surprising that DRGs were first developed for in-patient services. *Ambulatory Patient Groups* (APGs) are an American grouping system designed to analyse and compare the amount and type of resources used in ambulatory visits, much as DRGs do for inpatient services. So patients in each APG have similar clinical characteristics and similar resource use and cost. Like DRGs, APGs have a partitioning based on the presence of a significant procedure. 571 APGs are divided into 19 major ambulatory diagnostic categories based on body systems. There are two types of APGs; procedure and medical. Six data items are required to derive them: patient age, sex, diagnosis, procedure (if any), new or old problem and whether immediate admission was necessary. In the USA, APGs have been developed to analyse patient costs across the entire population, not just for Medicare patients, and aim to encompass the full range of ambulatory settings including some day surgery units, hospital emergency rooms and outpatient clinics. They are not designed to address phone contacts, home visits, nursing home services or inpatients.

However, the APG system fails adequately to separate different types of patients with corresponding levels of resource consumption. Contacts with radiologists, pathologists and some other professionals are excluded yet the cost of the tests is included with the total resources consumed.

Healthcare Resource Groups (HRGs) have been developed by the English National Casemix Office over the last two years as an alternative to DRGs, although are also HRGs intended to be both iso-resource and clinically homogeneous (NHSME 1993a). The main difference between DRGs and the HRGs is that the HRG grouper is speciality based and primarily driven by the procedure, if one has taken place. An automated grouper will analyse nationally recorded Körner information. It is expected that this will eliminate some of the statistical problems of DRGs and be more congenial to clinicians in England. Version 2 of the HRGs has been developed by clinical working groups, initiated in April 1993 and with the involvement of the Royal Colleges through the Joint Consultants' Committee and the Conference Information Group at all stages of the project. This version will allow records to be grouped into HRGs using ICD9 or ICD10 but not Read codes as these will be mapped from the ICD classifications and OPCS4.

Organising and managing coding

Classification and grouping systems are of little practical use unless the corresponding data about each patient are collected and recorded. Verbal entries in the patient's record have to be translated into the alphanumeric code(s) corresponding to the clinical classification(s) which apply, and these code(s) entered in the information system. This is no small task.

Traditionally, NHS coding has been organised in a centralised way with coding clerks based in the medical records department and accountable to the medical records manager. RHAs have trained coders and they implemented new classification and coding systems, in particular OPCS4. Quality assurance checks were also made in some regions on the data received from the Districts. Körner (DHSS 1982) recommended that:

1 Clinicians should record diagnostic data in medical notes in ways that would facilitate coding. A structured discharge summary was recommended.
2 Coding of diagnostic data should be carried out at local level so that those responsible have easy access to clinicians recording the data.
3 Training should continue to be given to those responsible for diagnostic coding. Adequate resources should be devoted to this task.

Unfortunately, many of these recommendations were not followed up and it is only in the last few years with the introduction of resource management and contracting that the coding process has become an issue of wide debate because, as Chapter 5 indicated, income may depend upon how efficiently it is done. Nowadays various models for managing coding are in operation, from having centralised coders to medical secretaries and consultants coding. The advantages and disadvantages of the three commonest models are as follows.

Centralised systems are the traditional organisation of the clinical coding function, employing clerical officers as part of the medical records function. These clerks were usually offered some basic training which was usually provided by the RHA. They were based in the medical records department and had no contact with the hospital medical staff. For a central system to work it is important to ensure that records are coded in a timely manner and any backlogs removed. The clinical information supplied to the coders has to be of a high standard and therefore some work has to be undertaken to improve the quality of this and the method of recording that information. It is also extremely important to ensure that the clinicians receive feedback. They should be supplied with routine information and the coders should be involved in discussions to improve the quality of the coded information. Advantages of centralised systems are that:

1 Experience of ICD is gained over many years by the clerks.
2 There is a central point to return case notes to, avoiding complicated administrative arrangements to ensure the notes are actually coded.
3 Validation of the patient's demographic and administrative details is easier, and this has assumed particular importance in contracting.
4 Some speciality based coding is possible in larger units.

Their disadvantages are:

1 Coders have no direct contact with clinicians, making quality difficult to monitor.
2 There is no clinical ownership of the information.
3 There is very little quality control or validation of diagnostic coding.
4 Information is not fed back to clinicians.

A decentralised model bases coding clerks alongside medical secretaries or on ward areas or in clinical directorates. Its advantages are that:

1 Coding clerks have access to the clinicians and can become more proficient in coding one speciality.
2 Records can be coded at the same time as a discharge summary is completed.
3 Good feedback to clinicians should help improve the quality of information.
4 If the coders are based on the ward all discharges can be coded prior to the discharge summary being completed and corrected if necessary at this point.

The disadvantages are:

1 Location of coding clerks in some hospitals could prove difficult, with space shortages.
2 Availability and numbers of coders may mean that some have to code across specialities or even directorates.
3 The coders feel isolated as they no longer have colleagues to discuss coding issues with.

Devolution of coding to medical secretaries is the third common model. This involves the coding being undertaken by the medical secretaries, usually as the discharge summaries are produced. It is more usually introduced when clinical workstations are, or with the introduction of the Read codes which exist as a computer file. It would be very unusual to find secretaries coding using ICD9 unless they have one of the automatic encoding products now available. The advantages of this system are that:

1 Medical secretaries work closely with the clinicians and will therefore be able to ask for assistance and advice when coding.
2 Notes will be coded as quickly as the discharge summaries are completed.
3 The consultants can have immediate feedback.

Disadvantages of this system are:

1 Training in coding systems and use of automatic encoders would have to be carried out.
2 The medical secretaries are unlikely to record co-morbidities which fall outside their speciality.
3 The medical secretaries will not check the patients' demographic and administrative details.
4 It may be necessary to increase the renumeration to medical secretaries.
5 Not all specialities complete discharge summaries so case notes may bypass the medical secretary.
6 Relief secretaries covering for holidays and sickness might not code.
7 The additional data required for obstetrics would not be collected by the medical secretaries.

It is essential that no matter who does the coding, training programmes are made available for them. This includes consultants, junior medical staff, coders, medical secretaries and also for those members of staff who use the coded information in the course of their work.

There is still the issue of quality verses quantity in clinical coding. Some trusts have decided to ensure 100 per cent coded data availability, often at the expense of good quality data. Data audit and validation of the codes and the consistency of their use should be routinely undertaken with validation mechanisms being built into the assignment of the Read codes. Without regular audit the quality and consistency of the information will not improve.

A study (Anon 1991–2) to evaluate the implementation of the Read codes in the Yorkshire Region suggests that however coding is organised, there has to be clinical involvement in it if the information produced is to be of a high quality. Although this study concerned Read codes its findings apply no matter what coding system is in use. The following benefits would probably arise from clinical involvement in any coding process:

1 Clinical ownership of the information because Read codes have to a large extent already achieved clinical acceptability.
2 Coding can be carried out for a wide range of patient characteristics not just for diagnoses and operative procedures.
3 Greater scope for development which allows changes in clinical practice to be taken into account and local requirements can also be addressed.

A considerable amount of work is required to ensure that the source documents from which the coding is carried out are appropriate for their purpose; but the information contained within those documents is still more vital to the success of the coding system. It is vital that clinicians accept their responsibility for producing clear diagnostic statements that can be coded. It is never the coders' responsibility to determine the main diagnosis or principal operation for a patient; their responsibility is to ensure the correct code is assigned. Once clinicians accept their responsibility for this and for ensuring that source documentation produced by junior medical staff is checked by a senior clinician the quality of coding will undoubtedly improve.

Chapter 10

MANPOWER DEVELOPMENT FOR NHS INFORMATION SYSTEMS

Lorraine Nicholson and Victor Peel

Health Information, training and education in the UK – a chequered history

The history of training and education for health information and technology has been one of recurrent difficulties and missed opportunities. There has been confusion between technology related training and information related training. Until quite recently, the need for skilled – but not necessarily expert – information staff has been small and the consequences of their failure have been minimal. Most important of all, prior to the health service reforms senior NHS managers have not taken this subject particularly seriously; if they have considered it to be important, they have not known what to do about it.

The context for health information and technology training in the 1970s might be represented by two camps: business systems managed by RHAs and innovative clinical computing led by small groups of interested clinical practitioners. These clinical professionals often produced and worked with single-user systems which required little training for other staff. At the same time, RHAs were recruiting and training in-house staff to do batch processing on large mainframe computers and they were relatively self-sufficient. The need to train staff across the whole NHS to collect and use information was not seen as an important issue. These skills were principally needed to support the formal planning process and an information discipline separate to the planning staff was not required. The capture of clinical information to be used for managerial purposes was rarely considered.

The early 1980s saw the creation of two groups which had related but separate briefs: the Körner Committee was to look at information requirements, while the National Computing Committee was to consider technological needs. This division of responsibility typifies the schizophrenia that bedevilled the NHS for a decade. The training of technologists was – and in some areas still is – seen as the highest priority in order that operational systems could be specified, acquired, installed and maintained in a cost-effective and well-organised manner. There is no reason to condemn this except that much of this work, and the training and education of the staff performing it, took place in splendid isolation from the growing awareness of the use of information among hospital, community and primary care staff and their demands for better access to useful clinical and management data which they could turn into relevant information.

With hindsight the work by Edith Körner and her colleagues can be seen to have underpinned subsequent moves to the general management concept and then the internal market. It is unfortunate that much of their initial logic and work was seen by the DHSS as making a stick to beat the NHS with: the resulting stick was called the 'Department of Health Central Returns'. There was little understanding of the need to train, let alone educate, staff whose main concern was information collection and analysis. This work was also largely focused at the DHAs' headquarters. By the late 1980s there were few staff with an information role in management positions in the community services, perhaps one or two in each unit. Their brief was to deliver the information for Department of Health Central Returns. This information was mainly centred around staff rather than patients and offered little opportunity to analyse the value of the work done by those staff. Things were not much better in general practice. At that time, the number of GP computer installations could be counted in handfuls; training was seen as teaching the practitioner and perhaps the receptionist how to operate a simple system.

As a result, there were few sponsors among senior management for information education or training processes at hospital level. Those of us who, in the mid–1980s, were encouraging senior staff to think through the need for clinically rich information systems often met with a stone wall of incomprehension. Any success by the NHS Training Authority (now the Training Directorate) in setting up education programmes for senior medical records managers in the late 1980s was achieved partly by good management but also in large part by gentle persuasion against the better judgement of some of those concerned. The NHS Training Authority undertook the first attempt to analyse the need for information and technology training in the mid–1980s. Their analysis distinguished between staff as users, providers or collectors of information (NHSTA 1985). A drawback to this analysis was that it emerged that many staff were involved in all three roles. Defining training and educational needs in practical situations was therefore difficult and developing ways to deliver that training was even more difficult.

Nevertheless, useful progress was made after lengthy consultation with the NHS. The consultation process was probably too long and another obstacle to success was that the service was being consulted about something that, at the time, it did not understand and which it did not see as a priority. The Department of Health and the NHS Training Directorate were therefore left to second-guess many local training needs.

As the Department of Health had not yet developed a formal information and IT strategy for England, staff had little understanding of what they were being trained to do and why they were doing it. It was not obvious what the natural progression between roles would be and how career paths in information work were structured. As a result, training initiatives were largely seen as short courses to transfer specific skills or the preparation of training material for local use.

The situation is potentially better in Scotland where, in 1989, a review of information-related training needs was commissioned which drew on many of the lessons provided by the earlier English study. The programme has since delivered a well-received information training initiative across Scotland. In Wales, the diagnostic phase has been completed and the service will soon begin piloting coordinated and integrated methods of delivering information training. In Northern Ireland the diagnosis of training needs has, so far, not been as comprehensive as work in the rest of the UK.

Despite the Resource Management Initiative, most of the technology staff working in the NHS in 1990 were still based in RHAs or DHAs and information staff were mostly based at the regions' main headquarters rather than in the regional computing centres. The value of medical records staff, who are at the heart of clinical data collection, was at last beginning to be recognised. This was partly because of the need to make sure that patient activity in hospitals was being counted accurately, and partly as a result of separate initiatives such as the programme to reduce waiting lists. The need to train staff to effectively code and classify clinical work was beginning to be appreciated. These activities have not been cheap. So far, around £20 million has been spent from central funds and probably half as much again has been provided locally.

Since 1990 there has been a marked improvement in the understanding of the needs of the NHS for training and development related to information and technology and that understanding is beginning to bear fruit. Investment in the Resource Management Initiative (RMI) has allowed large numbers of medical, nursing and management staff to understand more clearly why they need both clinical and management information and the consequences of not having it. A tremendous boost has been given to the Resource Management training programme by the health service reforms and the impact of the internal market on cost, quality and the combination in the price-performance ratio of service providers. It can be argued that, without the pressures of the internal market, many resource management training initiatives would have slowly but inexorably sunk out of sight. The purchase of HISSs has also required a breed of hospital based information staff. Five years ago the public health community – along with economists, clinicians, the caring professions and managers at purchasing and provider level – were giving little priority to information and the need for staff adequately trained and educated in the use of information. They have been drawn into the heart of the debate by the imperative to understand the health needs of the population, to be able to specify those needs and to be able to turn them into contracts for healthcare provision.

The healthcare market and the need to be able to specify and cost care in considerable detail, have been the agents of changing the agenda for NHS information training and education. There are now at least seven universities with centres in the UK which specialise in research, education and training in the medical or health information field. Most have a unique focus of interest: some are interested in the clinical-computer interface; some, like the authors' own, are particularly interested in the interplay between management and health information systems. Within this growing community of educators, a consensus is emerging as to who needs to be trained and for which roles. We are also closer to understanding what kind of education they will need before they are trained. Given the difficulties experienced with health and medical informatics over the last twenty years, few will believe that we have achieved this understanding until it has been demonstrated. In contrast to the millions already spent on training, the amount of money being centrally invested to create and promote this educational community is in the order of tens of thousands of pounds. It may well be that from these seeds will come the next generation of health information educators and trainers who will provide a bedrock of trained staff throughout the NHS which has so far been lacking. What will have to be done?

Occupational standards and professional training for health information staff

One way in which training can be developed for health information workers is by using a standards-based method. This section describes the method, illustrating it with the case of education and training for medical records staff. However the principles apply to the education and training of information staff of all kinds.

Occupational standards are statements of performance required of staff. At their simplest level they can be used as:

1 *Operational standards* to monitor the performance or quality of service of a whole department with reference to a particular activity, for example, reception or the maintenance of computer records.

2 As a *training objective* stating the performance level to be achieved after training.

3 An *assessment tool*, to assess staff performance after training.

For standards to be available as a training objective or assessment tool they first have to be generated, as an operational standard. Some general considerations apply to standards and standard-setting in almost any organisational context. Standards can be defined as 'agreed measures by which performance of achievement can be judged', or as in the *Concise Oxford Dictionary*:

> standard . . . serving as a basis for comparison . . . document specifying agreed properties for manufactured goods etc. . . . . degree of excellence etc. required for a particular purpose.

The standard-setting process is a dynamic one, as Figure 10.1 illustrates. Once standards have been set they must be used. It is more practical to use and evaluate a few standards regularly than large numbers of rarely used or evaluated standards which have no significant impact on the quality of service or performance. In order to be effective standards that are set must be both achievable and measurable. All the staff who work with them must be committed to the philosophy of achieving and then improving them as an ongoing process. Commitment to and ownership of the standards will only be attained by the involvement of everyone in the standard setting process. Quality circles provide the ideal forum to introduce this process and also to monitor and maintain the standards that have been set.

An example of how standards can be applied to a particular function is the *Compendium of Standards for Health Records* (NHSTD 1991). Current health services initiatives (service contracts, business plans, resource management, total quality management, medical audit) all require a positive response from the health records function, as they demand dramatically improved quantity and quality of information based on clinical data. Each highlights the critical importance of health records departments to the success of the organisation, and the need to invest in staff development and training.

Previously, training approaches in health records departments have concentrated on the role title. But job structures are changing in response to local needs and the implications of *Working for Patients* (Department of Health 1989a), becoming more diverse in different places. As these changes take place, and responsibility is increasingly delegated, a training approach which is based on traditional job titles is less and less useful. A competency-based approach to training gets round these difficulties by offering a set of standards of performance which can be used to help managers to identify the activities which need to be done, and the competences (including skills, knowledge and attitudes) required to perform them effectively. Managers have found that the traditional allocation of work between the different jobs

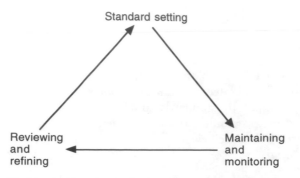

Figure 10.1   The standard setting cycle

of medical secretary, health records worker, clinical coder and receptionist may no longer be desirable. The competency-based approach identifies the functions and the different activities which have to be performed to provide support to clinicians in their clinical and management tasks. These functions can be identified as secretarial, health records management, waiting list management, clinical coding, audit, and reception of patients and visitors. As more trusts move towards a clinical directorate model of organisation and management, and medical records and secretarial staff are devolved to work in clinical support teams, the changes in job structure and content will become more marked. Managerial responsibility for staff is also being devolved and there is a corresponding increase in the requirement for consistent standards of performance across the boundaries of clinical directorates.

Part of the NHS Training Authority's (NHSTA; later the NHS Training Directorate) work in the health records field has been the development of a comprehensive compendium of standards of performance. These standards of performance form the basis of NHSTA's contribution to developing National Vocational Qualifications (NVQs) for administrative staff support-ing clinical work, but are being made available before the NVQs can be completed. At the same time, the standards are being tested in the NHS as part of a wider project concerning the training of ancillary and clerical staff. Guidance notes accompanying the *Compendium of Standards* show how they can be grouped in a variety of ways to suit local organisational needs and available staff resources (NHSTD 1991). Managers will then be able to use the standards to determine the learning and training resources to enable people to be trained to do the tasks which need doing at the level they need to be done. This means that the training provision required can be concentrated on the gap between what is already there and what is needed in each unit. Overstretched managers, who are already providing training and guidance to their staff 'on the job', will now be able to target their efforts.

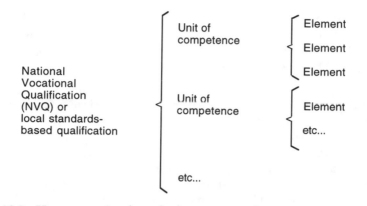

Figure 10.2   How occupational standards are structured

The standards contained within the *Compendium* were taken from the *Business Administration Standards* (developed by the administrative lead body for National Vocational Qualifications, the Management Charter Initative (MCI)) Management I and II Standards, standards developed specifically for clinical coding and extra units applicable to the health sector. The occupational standards for medical records staff comply with the format required of NVQs. The standards contained within the *Compendium* form the basis for the submission to the National Council for Vocational Qualifications. The *Compendium* can be used to provide the medical records manager and their staff with the means to develop an up to date training and assessment system rivalling that of any other industry or commerical concern. Occupational standards that are contained in *The Compendium of Standards for Health Records* all have a similar structure, shown in Figure 10.2.

The medical records department has been divided into a range of units of competence which are descriptions of large categories of work currently undertaken by the department. These are the units that staff undertaking training will have to demonstrate competence in. Jobs can be defined by clustering a number of units (together with their corresponding performance criteria or standards) which will describe the tasks that are required to be done. Each of the units, in turn, is broken down into a number of elements which describe aspects of the work. As an example Unit 1, which is concerned with filing, is subdivided into the two elements of:

1 file documents and open new files within an established filing system
2 identify and retrieve documents from within an established filing system.

Each of the elements in turn is broken down into a number of performance criteria or standards towards which a member of staff is trained and assessed. A member of staff trained and assessed as competent in all the performance criteria of each element is judged to have achieved competence in the overall unit.

Standards-based training should be as far as possible work based and easily accessible to everyone. It is accepted that existing staff and new staff may have to be approached differently. Training is relevant and appropriate for existing staff for three main reasons:

1 Jobs change and updating of skills is always important.
2 Some staff have never been trained properly having learned their jobs from other members of staff. By so doing they have learned some good habits and some not so good.
3 Existing staff are entitled to the opportunity to get access to training. This recognition has been sadly missing from medical records in the past with the exception of Association of Health Care Information and Medical Records Officers (AMRO) courses, which have not been made readily available to everyone.

At the same time, however, sensitivity must be shown to those staff who may be offended by the prospect of training after many years of service and see training as a threat, not an opportunity. So the introduction of standards-based training is best achieved by making it compulsory for all new staff but optional for existing staff.

The process for training new staff is essentially the same as for existing staff except that arrangements for assessing competence against each occupational standard will have to be undertaken during the first few weeks of work. Unlike an existing member of staff there will be no experience and observations of previous work. Activities that can be assessed initially for training purposes could include things like:

1 direct observation of work
2 use of spoken language in a variety of settings
3 legibility of written records
4 correctness of written records
5 response to other staff and supervision.

The assessment will also be work based and will be done in a way that encourages members of staff to identify their own training needs and to agree an action plan to address them.

Roles of national and international associations and organisations

Professional associations provide a forum for the exchange of ideas, concepts and developments within the profession. Their main objectives are to disseminate information and to share experiences through media such as conferences, workshops, seminars, professional journals and newsletters. Most professional associations provide a prescribed syllabus for study and professional examinations to provide a uniformly trained and qualified workforce. Membership categories vary from association to association but most provide membership opportunities to individuals or corporate bodies without the need to undertake the professional examinations. Some associations and organisations relevant to the development of health information staff are described briefly below but this is not an exhaustive list.

The *Institute of Health Services Management* (IHSM) is the leading professional body for health services management. The IHSM's major objectives are:

1 To promote excellence in health services management and the development of good managers.
2 To influence health services policy and its implementation.
3 To create and sustain a professional community of health service managers.

The IHSM offers qualifications which are tailor-made for those who manage, or want to manage, in the complex environment of health provision in the United Kingdom today. Membership of the IHSM provides recognition of professional status as a manager of health services. The IHSM is open to people at all levels and with different professional backgrounds. The Institute has a National Council which is made up of elected representatives from the Institute's 14 English Regions, coterminous with Regional Health Authorities, and the Scottish, Welsh and Northern Ireland Divisions. Each Region and Division has a programme of educational and social events including seminars, conferences and local links with other organisations. The categories of membership are: fellow or member (depending on educational qualifications), student or subscriber.

The *British Computer Society* (BCS) is concerned with information technology. It offers IT professionals the opportunity to participate in the development of their profession and a model for training and career progression. It offers computer users the ability to keep abreast of technical developments and to influence computing in their own profession. The BCS is incorporated by Royal Charter as the Professional Institution for Information Systems Engineering. It represents over 34 000 computer practitioners, more than any other society in Europe and it is a chartered engineering institution with the Engineering Council. As with all professional institutions, the BCS is concerned with maintaining and improving technical and ethical standards for the benefit of computing professionals and society at large. The Society is an authoritative voice to government and industry on all aspects of IT. It influences education through its own examinations, by accrediting degree and diploma courses, and by the planned training and career structure of the Professional Development Scheme. It influences legislation on data protection, safety, copyright, product liability and in other areas; and it provides experts for international standards committees and expert witnesses for courts and tribunals. The BCS provides up to date information through its technical journals, library, conferences and seminars.

It has 50 Specialist Groups covering key areas of the development and use of IT, and it is responsive to the need to set up new groups. Local branches provide contact with other members and direct involvement with the Society's work. The Young Professionals Group (for members agred 18–30) promotes the professionalism of young people in the IT industry and organises national and local meetings and conferences.

BCS membership categories include fellows, members and affiliateship (for professionals in disciplines other than computing), institutional membership, student and registrant membership. The BCS has members in all areas of the IT industry. (Further information can be obtained from: The British Computer Society, 13 Mansfield Street, London W1M OBP, Tel. 071 637 0471. Fax. 071 631 1049.)

In 1989, BCS helped form the *Council of European Professional Informatics Societies* (CEPIS) which is one route by which it gains access to the European Commission. CEPIS is committed to the single market through its 'Programme Europe' which focuses on key areas such as professional development, legal aspects, Eastern Europe and the demographic challenge.

The Association of Information Management and Technology Staff in the NHS (ASSIST) is a newly formed organisation for health information professionals. It provides networks for information exchange, activities and events at branch and national levels. It aims to influence national information policy, for instance by publishing research and other reports, to provide education and training and to raise professional standards through creating qualifications. Its membership categories are ordinary, honorary and retired membership. Further details may be obtained from the Membership Officer, ASSIST, PO Box 1022, Bristol BS99 1BF. Work on a national statement of recognition for information management and technology staff started in 1993 and is due to be piloted in 1994–5.

The *World Health Organisation* (WHO) is a specialised agency of the United Nations with primary responsibility for international health matters and public health. Through this organisation, which was created in 1948, the health professions of some 165 countries exchange their knowledge and experience. By means of direct technical cooperation with its member states, and by stimulating such cooperation among them, WHO promotes the development of comprehensive health services, the prevention and control of diseases, the improvement of environmental conditions, the development of health manpower, the coordination and development of biomedical and health services research, and the planning and implementation of health programmes. Progress towards better health throughout the world also demands international cooperation in such matters as establishing international standards for biological substances, pesticides, and pharmaceuticals; formulating environmental health criteria; recommending international non-proprietary names for drugs; administering the International Health Regulations; revising the *International Classification of*

Diseases, Injuries, and Causes of Death (WHO 1992; see Chapter 9); and collecting and disseminating health statistical information. Further information on many aspects of WHO's work is presented in the Organisation's publications. The World Health Organisation's headquarters are in Geneva, Switzerland, its European Regional Office in Copenhagen.

The *Association of Health Care Information and Medical Records Officers* (AMRO) was founded in 1948 at the Christie Hospital in Manchester and now has members throughout Great Britain, its main aim being to provide professional guidelines and support for persons working in health records, information and patient services. At national level workshops, conferences and seminars are arranged at regular intervals and advice is provided to members on current professional issues and legal matters. At local level there are 18 regional branches organising educational, training and social events for members and it is one of these branches which hosts the national conference each year. The conference aims to provide delegates with an insight into new developments in the NHS as well as keeping them informed of developments in the medical records profession overseas. AMRO is an examining body organising its own examinations in Great Britain and overseas for its student members. The examinations cover such subjects as medical records services and management, anatomy and physiology, statistics, personnel and general management and medical terminology and classification.

The publication of *Working for Patients* (Department of Health, 1989a) and its subsequent implementation has made many changes in health records with a greater emphasis on the quality of patient care and the requirement to collect more detailed information on individual patients for contracting and future planning of the service. AMRO accredits educational establishments that provide taught courses to enable students to take the associations professional examinations. It has produced a *Handbook for Quality Control in Medical Records* (AMRO 1985) which enables managers to assess the quality of their service and monitor it in an ongoing way. AMRO publishes a professional journal which is circulated quarterly to members and subscribers. The *AMRO Journal* publishes high quality articles relating to current medical records practice, educational developments and reports from branches. Its membership categories are affiliate membership, licentiateship, fellow, student and certificate membership. Further information about AMRO can be obtained from: The AMRO Office, Pear Tree Cottage, Mill Lane, Horsemans Green, Whitchurch, Shropshire SY13 3EA. Tel. 0948 74573.

AMRO is a member organisation of the *International Federation of Health Records Organisations* (IFHRO) and has a Director to the Grand Council of the Federation. IFHRO has the following objectives:

1 To provide a means of communication between persons working in the field of health records in the various countries of the world.

2 To advance the standards of health records in hospitals, dispensaries, and other health and medical institutions.
3 To promote and/or develop techniques for efficient use of health records for patient care, statistics, research, teaching and to disseminate these among member organisations.
4 To provide means for the exchange of information on education requirements and training programmes for health records in all countries.

IFHRO was established in 1968 to bring together national associations which had been formed to improve health or medical records keeping practices in their countries. Health records organisations in the following countries are active members of the Federation (1988):

Australia	Jamaica	Philippines
Britain	Japan	South Korea
Canada	Kenya	USA
France	Netherlands	Venezuela
Germany	New Zealand	
Israel	Nigeria	

These national associations recognised the need to have a permanent organisation to exchange information internationally in the health records field. IFHRO is a non-profit-making body representing the health records profession. The Federation is invited to WHO sponsored meetings and it works closely with WHO on specific projects which have been identified as of particular concern to WHO in the field of health records. These include education of health record keepers; health records needs in developing countries; legislation concerning health records. IFHRO's educational activities are aimed at improving health care through the development of good health recording practices. In this regard IFHRO complements the work of WHO and is only limited in its effectiveness by finance. Communication between active and associate members is encouraged through the *International Health Records Newsletter* published five times a year and made available to all members. Contributions are invited from individuals in member organisations. The editorial address is: Linda Bergen, 876 Gainsway Road, Yardley, PA 19067, USA.

There are two basic categories of member: active and associate. Active membership is composed of one national organisation per country of persons working in the field of health records, associate membership is available to an individual working in the field of Health Record Science in a country where there is no national organisation eligible for active membership in the Federation. Associate member subscription is US$10 a year. Individuals in any country, including those whose organisations are active members, can support IFHRO as Friends. Each Friend receives a personal copy of the International Health Records Newsletter by air mail. Friends subscribe minimum rates as shown above plus any extra they can afford to support IFHRO publications. Further information about IFHRO can be obtained from the secretary/treasurer, Phillip Roxborough, 2/365 Richardson Road, Mount Roskill, Auckland 4, New Zealand.

The *National Coding Reference Centre* is a new organisation which is being established in response to an identified need within the NHS. Its purpose is to establish national standards and definitions for clinical coding. The centre has been established by NHS Information Systems (NHSIS) and is funded initially by the Resource Management Unit of the NHS Management Executive. All of the regional clinical coding tutors (14 from England, one from Wales, one from Northern Ireland) will be participating in the work of the Centre. Working groups will report to the Executive Director of NHSIS, who will report to the Committee for the Review of Information Requirements (CRIR), who will grant formal approval for change. Dissemination of information from the Centre will be through the clinical coding tutors.

Chapter 11

PROCURING HEALTHCARE INFORMATION SYSTEMS

Caroline Rae and Roger Dewhurst

Introduction

Choosing and procuring information systems (IS) and information technology (IT) has traditionally been the preserve of the IT specialist. At this stage the manager often withdraws; the business objectives have been identified, the information strategy developed, and now what are needed are the tools to do the job. These tools are understood by the IT specialist and thus the task of acquiring them has largely been their role. These tools – the information systems – are a key element in supporting the business. They are the means by which the benefits to the organisation, which have been identified as part of the business strategy, can be delivered.

Since the middle 1980s the NHS has increasingly recognised the value of project management techniques for the procurement, installation and implementation of IT systems. With the introduction of the purchaser–provider split the procurement of IT has, often for the first time, become the direct responsibility of individual provider units or DHAs.

Why should generalist managers take the lead in the choice and procurement of IT systems? Certainly, expert advice is required to tackle the many and complex technical issues but the choice and procurement of IT is an extension of the process which the organisation has already begun. It involves the more precise definition of information and facilities required by users – extending the analysis undertaken as part of the production of an information strategy. It also involves more than the procurement of a piece of technology. The products and services associated with the technology are varied and their suppliers operate in different ways. The range of products and services purchased under the broad heading of information systems will impact on many aspects of the life of the organisation.

Making choices based on a consideration of so many different factors can, however, be made more difficult by the complexity of the technical issues that may be involved. Recently, the Audit Commission has focused attention on the effective management of the procurement process. In their 1992 report they state:

> A new generation of purchasers of IT has been created in DHAs, Trusts, FHSAs and GP Fundholders and, generally speaking, many of the officers concerned are unfamiliar with established practices of procuring and managing an IT service. Whilst spending on IT is increasing, auditors have found little evidence that it is well managed and well controlled ... it is essential that there are safeguards against the possibility of effectiveness being reduced through unco-ordinated development. (Audit Commission 1992)

This chapter is designed to help guide non-IT specialists who have direct or indirect responsibility for managing the IT and information systems procurement. It is not a 'teach yourself IT manual'. Its purpose is to help managers identify what they need to know, what issues they should be aware of, what kind of advice and support they should be looking for, where to look and what sort of behaviours and techniques to expect. The chapter is also written for those senior managers who have empowered the procurement process but have delegated the authority for its completion. If you do not know what you are looking at how can you recognise when a good job is being done and support the people doing the job on your behalf?

The purchase of a complete computer system can be broken down into a number of components:

1 Application software, discussed in the next section.
2 Software used to build the application, also discussed briefly in the next section.
3 Selection of hardware manufacturers' language compilers; and
4 Choice of an operating system.
5 Hardware procurement. This, and the previous two components are outlined in section 3 of this chapter.

The remainder of the chapter then outlines the procurement process itself.

Procuring application software

Application software is the most important element of an information system. Organisations only buy computers to run software applications which support their businesses. Application software can be developed by the individual organisation. This closely tailors it to the organisation's requirements but is likely to be a lengthy process requiring more skills within than many organisations have. It is unlikely that an individual organisation would wish to develop a complete patient administration system in-house, using its own resources, generally it will look to purchase a patient administration system that has been developed by a commercial supplier for widespread use within the NHS. In the NHS there has been a move away from bespoke applications towards 'off the peg' turnkey application software.

A third alternative is the collaborative development of application software between supplier and individual organisation. This option has proved popular in areas of business development which are new, for example the development of CMMSs at the beginning of the Resource Management Initiative. However, it requires considerable and sustained commitment from both organisations and a clear and concise view of user requirements from the purchasing organisation. Whatever the approach taken to the procurement of application software, it is essential to have a clear, comprehensive statement of user requirements. Without this it will be impossible to judge whether the software meets your needs.

In the course of this chapter it is not possible to outline a comprehensive list of application software that is commonly in use within the NHS today. However, the following list is a selection of the most commonly used applications in the NHS with a brief note of the criteria by which software might be selected.

Patient administration system (PAS)

What a patient administration system contains is explained Chapter 5. A first criterion by which to evaluate a registration module and master patient index is whether other systems can share the index, or do they have patient indices of their own? If the latter is the case, how are separate indices kept in step? Does this involve duplicate effort in capturing information or are there automatic mechanisms for transferring information? Secondly one must ask what the quality of the index is? For example, does it contain duplicate records for the same patient? Are key items of information captured accurately, for example details of the patient's GP and the postcode of their address are essential in deciding who is responsible for commissioning the treatment? Can records be traced using a patient's NHS number? (This will become important in future.)

An inpatient management module should assist in the effective use of hospital resources, as explained in Chapter 5. Criteria by which to evaluate inpatient modules are, first, how far can they be used, with other systems, for prospective planning and scheduling of resources? Obviously, where patients are admitted immediately and not from a waiting list, this is not feasible.

However, if this module is linked to those supporting the planning and scheduling of outpatient appointments and the management of waiting lists, such prospective planning should be possible.

Unfortunately, many systems do not allow this; rather, they support the collection of information as a patient is admitted, discharged or transferred between wards or into the care of another clinician and provide retrospective management information. Secondly, one must consider how accessible and useful is the information for day-to-day, hour-by-hour, management? Is the module only concerned with workload recording for subsequent use in monitoring progress within contracts? This may reflect whether the system can be accessed from wards, diagnostic departments and clinicians' offices.

Criteria by which to evaluate outpatient modules include whether they allow information to be recorded on the treatment provided? As more procedures are undertaken in outpatient clinics, rather than on wards as day cases or inpatients, this will become important. Already the contracting process requires a hospital to be able to identify under which contract a particular appointment is being paid for but better information will be required if different prices are to be charged for appointments involving procedures rather than assessment or review of the patient's condition. The problems of collecting this information are associated with the large numbers of appointments. Where procedures are planned this may best be captured at the time of booking when it can be used for resource scheduling. Unfortunately, the design of many systems does not currently allow this. Secondly, one should check whether the outpatient and inpatient management modules are linked to allow prospective planning of the treatment to be provided to an individual patient?

Order Communications and Results Reporting modules do not form part of the portfolio of traditional PAS modules. They are however a key element of fully integrated patient care systems. Often, in order to introduce this type of system it is necessary to replace an existing patient administration system with such an integrated product. These modules allow clinicians, nurses and other authorised staff to order tests and diagnostic procedures, medications and supplies via computer terminals located where patients are being treated and transfer these orders or requests electronically to the departments who provide the tests or supplies. This type of module facilitates communication and also allows the departments to record when a test has been undertaken and its results. These details can then be accessed by clinicians and nurses on wards, in their offices and in clinics. The benefits of these systems include: preventing duplicate orders; reducing the clerical effort for professional staff and releasing time for direct patient care; speeding up the communications process for test results; and better use of stocks.

As these systems are costly a key issue in their introduction is the identification of these benefits and a clear programme involving all relevant staff to realise them. Often the benefits can only be realised if healthcare professionals are prepared to change their existing working practices. With the introduction of an integrated set of systems, involving an extensive network of terminals, it is possible to introduce other functions, including the tracking of patients case notes. The benefits of this are associated with increased productivity of medical records, nursing and clerical staff.

A key issue with all departmental systems (see Chapter 5) is whether they are patient based and are integrated or interfaced with the PAS master patient index. Where departmental systems have their own patient indices with independent referencing or numbering, it can be difficult to build up a picture of the total package of care provided to an individual patient.

This brings us to the various management information systems that are available.

Case mix management systems (CMMSs)

CMMSs are systems which allow analysis of the services provided to patients and the resources used to support planning and monitoring of both the hospitals overall business plan and individual clinical directorates' 'business plans'. The systems were introduced as part of the national Resource Management Initiative. The logic and purpose of these systems are discussed more fully in Chapters 2 and 5, which also indicate what basic analyses CMMSs should be able to perform. CMMSs should allow clinicians and managers to answer questions about the types of patients treated (the term 'case mix' refers to groups of patients with similar conditions requiring similar treatment); the treatment actually provided to patients; and the resources used.

Medical audit systems

Medical audit systems are designed to support individual clinicians in recording and analysing the treatment they provide to patients. Again at the heart of these systems, which are generally microcomputer based, is a database of patients and individual care events. One potential problem with the widespread use of these stand-alone systems is that the information collected in them by individual clinicians differs from that available in corporate systems, either because of different definitions or lack of completeness (in either system). A key issue is therefore the integration of these systems with the main patient-based hospital systems. Often, medical audit systems, as well as providing clinicians with the ability to retrospectively analyse the treatment provided to patients and its outcome, contain operational features such as waiting list management.

GP systems

GP systems (see Chapter 4) are available from over 100 separate suppliers although the market is dominated by four or five firms. The systems support GPs in managing both the clinical and financial aspects of their practices, allowing them to maintain patient records, record and generate prescriptions, generate claims for payment and monitor and maintain fundholding budgets. To date there have been few common standards among GP systems. With the introduction of fundholding, systems must comply with a national specification for certain functions. NHSME will issue a minimum specification for GP systems, compliance with which will form the basis for increased reimbursement towards the purchase of such systems (see also Chapters 4 and 12).

FHSA computer systems

FHSA computer systems are also described in Chapter 4. Currently, all FHSAs use the same standard national application software to support their business activities. This software allows the FHSAs to maintain a register of all patients registered with GPs within their area and to process contracted claims for payment made by GPs in respect of the services they provide. The register provides a limited source of information for local primary care service planning. Currently, the FHSA system is being redeveloped to provide better performance, as Chapter 4 explains.

HISS systems

HISS systems (see Chapter 5) are the subject of recent central guidance on procurement. These frameworks assist HISS purchasers in identifying suppliers whose systems meet specific functional requirements and whose suppliers are judged to meet basic performance and reliability criteria. HISS purchasers who use this guidance benefit from a much simplified procurement process, having a smaller number of proven suppliers to chose from and be able to concentrate on specific local tailoring requirements. Following the guidance incidentally shortens the tendering process as doing so also completes many of the steps required by EU-GATT procedures (see 6 below). Several potential purchasers of HISS systems are forming purchasing consortia in order to pool knowledge and expertise while still allowing local tailoring of the systems. Similar developments are beginning among purchasers of other types of healthcare information system.

Besides application software of any of the above kinds, it will also be necessary to procure supporting software to 'build' the application. Often the purchase of a complete system will involve the purchase of separate licences for different software products which have been used to develop the application. This is particularly the case if it is intended to undertake further development work in-house, even if this development is only the preparation of new reports or *ad hoc* enquiries of the information held within the application. Typically, these software products include (first) database management software, relational databases such as Oracle, Ingres and Infomix, and reporting and analysis software. 'Fourth generation' application development and enquiry tools may be part of the product set of the database management software. It may also be necessary to purchase a language compiler and libraries from the hardware manufacturer. The application's operating system must also match the operating system software for the chosen hardware (see the following section; and Chapter 1). Historically, hardware manufacturers developed their own proprietary operating system software products exclusive to their range of computers. For example, ICL's VME or IBM's VM/CMS environments were exclusive to those manufacturers' range of products. Applications in these environments were often not available on other manufacturers' hardware. Now the majority of manufacturers offer hardware using operating systems which comply to common 'Posix' standards (Chapter 1 explains what operating systems and standards are). Increasingly, the same application is available on a range of different hardware manufacturers' products. This brings us to the selection of hardware to run the chosen applications on.

Procuring computer hardware

Selection of the most appropriate computer hardware, operating system software, communications hardware and software, is obviously an important factor in the successful implementation of application software.

The hardware which has to be selected includes the computer processor or processors, which run both the operating systems software and the software products used to build the application. It is also necessary to select the peripheral devices connected to these computer processors. Any computer system will have a range of devices connected to its processors. Typically these devices include, first, disc devices, for the storage of data and programmes. The price of disc storage has decreased significantly in recent years and a range of new types of device such as optical discs has become available (see Chapters 1 and 8). Tape devices are typically used for the distribution of software from suppliers, to back up the application data and programs onto, and to receive or transfer information to other organisations or computer systems. Again, the range of tape devices, the volume of data that can be stored on the tapes and the speed with which information can be transferred to and from the tapes has changed significantly in recent years. Within the NHS a significant amount of information is still transferred between organisations on half-inch magnetic tapes. However for the other purposes outlined above, digital audio tapes or other forms of compact tape cartridges which will contain high volumes of data (such as exabyte tapes) are increasingly used.

The printers required will depend on the application and the business areas which they are supporting. These will determine whether or not high quality output is required and the volumes of bulk printing that will be undertaken. The type of terminal or workstation required will also depend on the application and the tasks that individual users are required to perform. Some users may only require 'dumb' or unintelligent terminals, which have no processing capacity of their own while others may require personal computers to act as terminals or workstations because some of the processing takes place at their terminal. In both cases one of the key issues to be considered is whether or not the terminals or workstations will need to be linked to other computer processors running separate applications.

There may be no advantage in purchasing the complete range of peripheral devices required to run an application from the same source as the computer processor. Given the substantial discounts available within the NHS because of nationally agreed purchasing arrangements, it may be cheaper to purchase IBM items such as personal computers to act as workstations. If such an approach is taken, it is obviously important to establish agreed standards for the separately purchased peripherals with both the supplier of the application and the supplier of the computer processors and to ensure that appropriate maintenance and support arrangements are in place (see below). Communications hardware will be required to provide the connections between remotely located peripherals and processors, and hence communications software to provide facilities to access different processors across a network and to manage the connection of peripheral devices to these processors. Communications software will have to support both terminal emulation (the direct access of an application running on a particular processor from either a dumb terminal or a personal computer acting as a workstation) and file transfer between storage devices and printers connected across the network.

In specifying the hardware requirements of any particular application, a number of key issues need to be considered when specifying the overall operational requirement and in subsequent discussions with potential suppliers.

The basic sizing issue to consider is whether the overall hardware configuration, including storage devices for data, will support the application being used to its full extent. Obviously the configuration of computer processors needs to be sufficiently powerful to provide the performance required by users. Also the storage devices must have sufficient capacity to allow for existing volumes of data and any expected future growth in volumes. The specification of numbers of devices needs to take into account that generally disks do not operate efficiently when used to full capacity and to allow sufficient space for any overheads associated with the design of the application, in particular file indices to allow rapid access. The storage capacity defined will also need to take into account requirements for periodic reorganisation of files and the retrieval of archived information.

What is required will depend on the nature and design of the application. It is important to ask the potential systems suppliers to explain how they have arrived at a particular configuration. It will be necessary to supply them with information to enable them to estimate the volumes of data the application will need to accommodate. Information is also required on the numbers of users that can be expected to be accessing the information at any point in time and the sorts of task that these users will be undertaking. The suppliers' response should indicate, for example, how the volumes of data are to be stored and whether any particular tables or files are critical to the performance of the application. The suppliers should also indicate whether the size of the central processor is critical to performance or whether the speed with which information can be retrieved from disks is as, or more, important.

The expected reliability of the overall system being purchased can be expressed as a series of measures which indicate the proportion of the time for which the system is potentially unavailable, or is likely to be inoperable for a variety of reasons. The system may not be available because of problems with the application software; the operating system software; the communications software and hardware; the communications network; the processors; the peripheral devices; or because of other factors such as planned maintenance. In the last five areas, steps can be taken in specifying an initial configuration to support the application which will minimise the potential for the system becoming inoperable. The basic issue to be considered is how the organisation's business will be affected if the system, or parts of it are not working. Key questions are:

1 How long can the organisation manage without certain of the application functions?
2 What procedures can be put in place to minimise disruption if the system is unavailable?
3 How long will it take to recover from a full or partial failure of the system?

There are a number of health service applications where high levels of reliability are essential. In specifying hardware configurations in these instances there may be a need to consider multiple processors to support the application and mirrored data storage devices. The communications network topography needs to ensure that failure in one part of the network does not lead to its total unavailability. Clearly, there are costs associated with the requirement for high levels of reliability.

An important issue that should not be overlooked in purchasing a computer system is the environment in which the processors and certain peripherals are going to be located. While the processors which support many smaller applications may not require siting in specially prepared locations, it is important to establish whether or not any changes are required to accommodate additional air conditioning, temperature control or protection from adjacent electronic equipment. Factors that ought explicitly to be considered are:

1 The weight of the proposed equipment and its impact on floor loadings within the building.
2 The clearances required around the processor and any particular peripherals.
3 The temperature and humidity conditions required by the hardware, particularly the processors.
4 The heat that will be produced by a particular configuration and how this can be controlled.
5 Any special lighting conditions required.
6 The noise levels associated with the hardware, especially printers.
7 Requirements for control of dust.
8 Power supply requirements.

In addition, the need to maintain a secure environment for confidential information should be taken into account.

Implementation and training support

Services which you may consider procuring as part of your total package include implementation support, maintenance and ongoing system support.

The issues you may wish to consider in procuring implementation and training will be influenced both by your own organisation and its skills and the nature of the system which you are procuring. For example, you may choose one particular package if you are purchasing a small operational system, a different package for a hospital-wide operational system and yet a third package for a system which will have a limited number of users, such as a management information system, but which will have a big impact on the strategic management of your organisation.

The first decision you will have to make is whether you wish to see your system delivered by your supplier in as short a time as possible or whether you wish the process to be a longer one with the supplier and yourselves working jointly on installation and implementation. The essential difference is whether you are procuring the support of a supplier to install the system (that is where a system is technically functioning but not necessarily being used widely on a day-to-day basis) or whether you wish to contract for installation and implementation, where the suppliers remain heavily involved with you until the system is being widely used. There are significant price differences in the two approaches and the control mechanisms which you will wish to use, both within the contract and throughout your two organisations, will differ.

The advantage of procuring for installation only is that it is easier to define than the total installation and implementation process, has obvious start and end points and it is easier to see whether the supplier has done a good job. As it is an easily defined process, suppliers may give you a more accurate idea of both cost and the timescales involved and any problems incurred are likely to be more readily identified. However, a disadvantage of installation support alone is that the skills and expertise that the suppliers have built up in using the system are not easily transferred to your staff. More importantly perhaps is that the supplier's main obligation lies in ensuring that the system functions and performs successfully. Installation implies more than simple delivery of the system and will require you to undertake acceptance testing which is agreed with the supplier during procurement. The critical difference between installation and implementation is that the latter process ensures not only that the system performs but that it is used effectively within your organisation.

It is often difficult for an organisation implementing a system fully to determine its tailoring requirements during installation, before the system has been in use for a while. In such circumstances the implementation period can be a critical time for the supplier and users to clarify final requirements. Equally, when suppliers are involved in the implementation of a system, rather than its mere installation, they will be keen to ensure that the momentum is kept going within the unit and that continued attention and effort is focused on implementation. Finally, suppliers providing implementation support can bring experience from other organisations who have used the product. This experience, however, may also be gained through the support of user groups (for further discussion of this see the section on maintenance and ongoing support). In considering the type of support you require you will also have to decide whether you need it solely for the technology itself or whether you are looking to extend support to its widespread application and its use within the unit.

Thus the first decisions to be made concern the overall approach to implementation which you wish to share with the supplier. Then there are further matters to consider.

The first concerns the management of the implementation process. It is likely that both you and the supplier will wish to appoint project managers to oversee the installation and implementation of the system. This should be clarified together with the relative position of the project managers within both organisations. For the supplier who is sub-contracting some of the work to other suppliers, it is necessary to consider whether there will be one project manager on behalf of the supplier who will be responsible for all input to the project or whether project managers will also be appointed for the subsidiary suppliers. The former approach has the advantage that there is one individual with whom you have to deal who takes total responsibility for the work carried out by the supplier. The advantage of the latter approach is that it is possible to talk directly to the sub-contractors who will have the specialist knowledge of their own areas of work and issues may therefore be tackled more quickly.

Secondly, the approach taken to project management must be agreed and it is important to state whether it is intended to use any specific project management methodology, for example PRINCE (see Chapters 1 and 7). Either way, it is also important to clarify the project management structure, the existence of any project team and subsidiary working parties, who will be represented upon them and to whom these teams will be accountable, what the commitment of each side is to managing the installation and implementation processes and what resources each organisation is committing. Besides identifying the individuals and methodology, we strongly recommend that a project plan be produced. This plan may be drawn up by you or by the supplier on their own but is more likely to be realistic if both parties draw it up, committing themselves to the dates and resources stated within the project plan. The individuals working on the project must be experts well qualified to carry out the roles that they have been assigned, and must also work well as a team and get on together.

The implementation and installation process is as critical to the successful introduction of your system as the choice of system itself. As part of the procurement process you may wish to meet representatives of the suppliers who may join your installation and implementation team. Although it is advisable to seek clarification on the type of skills the supplier may wish to assign to the project, it is unlikely that during the procurement process the supplier will be able to name individuals working at each stage of the project. Assurances are required that the individuals who will be assigned to you are of the same degree of expertise as those who you have met during the course of procurement, or even that the individuals you have already met will continue to participate beyond the procurement process into installation or implementation. Successful implementation of information system depends heavily on the strength of the partnership between purchaser and supplier. Clear roles and lines of communication are essential for success.

Deciding on the extent to which you want your supplier to provide training support for your system is very similar to the issues to be taken into account when considering implementation. Either the supplier is given total responsibility or the skills are passed to a core group of in-house staff who take the responsibility for extending training throughout the organisation.

If the supplier will provide all training it becomes necessary to identify precisely during procurement the numbers and types of staff and the training they will require. A whole hospital or a communications system, for instance, may require the training of many hundreds of ward based and non-ward based staff. Training at the right time and location by an outside supplier may be costly and difficult for the supplier to synchronise with system implementation. It may, however, be a better solution where training in specialised technologies would be particularly beneficial.

The alternative approach to training is some form of in-house provision with in-house 'core trainers' who would be trained by the system supplier and then continue the training for the system internally. This enables you to schedule the training as and when required by your users and provide refresher courses as often as necessary. It may also be cheaper. However, you must ensure that the core trainers keep their skills up to date (they may need refresher training from the supplier as changes are made to the system). Physical facilities for training would have to be provided by you, normally on site.

The different types of training which may be required are system training (technical training about application software); training specific to your application software; knowledge-based training (e.g. 'how to do it' training, training in using the system and its benefits); and awareness training for staff who may not necessarily be directly affected by the system but who need to have an awareness of what is taking place and why. It is also necessary to decide how to:

1 Provide the facilities required.
2 Identify the numbers of training staff required and their own training and development needs.
3 Identify training needs including refresher training.
4 Provide continuing training support (such as the support for an on-site help line or a central point for the referral of questions of operation of the system to the system supplier).
5 Free staff from their duties to enable them to attend the training programme.
6 Define training course delivery with the supplier – is this to be by the number of training hours delivered or by the number of staff trained in the particular aspects of use of the system?
7 Monitor the effectiveness of training delivery approaches.

Maintenance and ongoing support

As part of the procurement of your information system, you will also have to consider procuring maintenance and ongoing support services. Suppliers differ in the type of cover that they can offer but you should consider what degree of support you require as follows.

Hardware support may prove a problem where the supplier of your system supplies a system hardware that they themselves do not manufacture. You will wish to consider whether you wish hardware support to be provided by a systems supplier, perhaps under a facilities management contract (see below), or whether you wish to contract directly with the hardware supplier for support. In deciding upon the support you require, consider what response times you feel to be acceptable, what hours of cover, the location of your support team and what back up facilities will be necessary. For servicing peripheral devices or less critical areas of the system, the use of third parties, supplying neither the system nor the hardware, for servicing, may be appropriate.

With *systems software* as with hardware, the supplier of your information system might be using proprietary systems software. You will again need to decide whether to contract directly with the supplier of this software for your support. You will need to clarify, under any support contract, policy regarding updated software, newly released versions of the software and the support desk facilities.

In the section on implementation we looked at the tailoring of the application software that may be necessary to make it suit the particular requirements of your organisation. In deciding the necessary level of *day-to-day support* one must first identify the degree to which immediate support for users of the system is required (for example whether they need to be able to contact a support desk manned by the systems supplier) and what the expected performance would be in correcting faults once reported.

In the course of running the system, further changes will be needed and it is important to establish in any support contract the degree to which it is possible for these to be carried out in-house. For example, can code tables, archiving routines or standard reporting routines be tailored by your in-house support staff or would it be necessary to go to the systems supplier to have these minor amendments made? If you feel it necessary to have more major changes made to the software, it is important to establish whether, if these are carried out in-house, the supplier will support you in the future should problems occur with your software. A supplier using a standard support contract will probably wish to restrict the types of changes that can be made to the software in-house. Major changes to the software may mean that future updated versions of the software may be difficult to instal on your system and this needs to be clarified before any support contract is taken out. Clarification will also be needed, particularly on jointly developed software, on the status of copyright and licensing of the application software.

Additionally, you will need to consider the *policy* regarding either updated software or new versions or releases of the software. Updated software releases are designed to deal only with minor changes that the supplier wishes to make to the software, perhaps to incorporate changes in legislation or screen design changes made in response to user suggestions, for example. New versions of the software embody more major changes to the content of the software, perhaps new features or an extended or changed database. It is important to clarify whether the software support contract would cover the implementation and installation of either updates or new versions of the

software. Looking to the future development of the software in the medium
to long term, you should establish with the supplier how suggestions from
you, the user, may be incorporated in any future software development. For
example, some suppliers support user groups where not only common
problems and solutions can be shared, but also both minor and long-term
developments of the software can be identified and agreed upon by
representatives of the users of the software.

Maintenance and ongoing support will be required to tackle both
day-to-day problems and medium to long-term problems as well as required
developments of the system. This support is most likely to be provided by a
combination of in-house staff and one or more suppliers although either
party individually may provide the service. Roles and responsibilities need to
be defined clearly.

Total supplier support could be provided through a facilities management
arrangement where, for example, the staff providing both day-to-day and
long-term development are provided by the supplier on your site (or,
alternatively, on the supplier's site), and where the hardware and systems
software may also be located either with you or with the supplier. A further
option is to use a bureau service for the provision of the system, both
hardware and software, where the software is not exclusively owned by the
organisation but used by them in conjunction with many other organisations.

Managing procurement

The process of procuring information systems should be designed to
demonstrate objectivity and fairness to suppliers, as well as ensuring that the
solution most appropriate to the requirements of the procuring organisation
is selected. The main drawback of a formal procurement process is often seen
as being the time it takes. For both the purchaser and the supplier,
unnecessary delays and effort are costly and in the end the price will reflect
them. In undertaking a procurement, it is critical that all parties understand
the importance of deadlines and responsibilities. For a major procurement,
the use of a structured project management methodology such as PRINCE to
manage the process is beneficial (see Chapters 1, 2 and 7). Not only does a
methodology provide an environment more likely to ensure that the project is
successful. It also provides a structure within which to identify decision
points and develop documentation.

The NHS Supplies Authority, with the support of the NHSME and the
suppliers of information system has launched POISE – Procurement of
Information Systems Effectively. POISE consists of guidelines on best practice and a set of standard procurement stages and tools. Its aim is to ensure
greater consistency in procurement, especially the importance of defining the
business case for the systems investment and the benefits expected at the

outset, of following public procurement rules and good practice and of allowing suppliers flexibility in proposing solutions to a clearly defined business need. It also emphasises the fair, consistent evaluation of suppliers throughout procurement and the need to minimise NHS and supplier costs by using a consistent process. POISE identifies 19 separate steps in procurement, divided into four basic stages in procurement.

The first POISE stage is planning the procurement, involving:

Step 1:   Initial appraisal to state the business case for the planned investment, explicitly identifying the benefits which will justify the costs.

Step 2:   Initial market survey to identify what potential solutions are available.

Steps 3, 4 and 5: Planning the procurement, agreeing budgets, timescales and how to comply with legislation and standing orders, and establishing a formal project management structure.

The second POISE stage is the preparation of various documents for use during the procurement. All should be formally approved by the Project Board. This involves;

Step 6:   Prepare a detailed statement of need (DSON), representing the detailed operational requirement mentioned earlier.

Step 7:   Summarising the DSON, noting mandatory requirements which suppliers proposed solutions must meet. This is the 'statement of need'.

Step 8:   Production of the EU advertisement.

Step 9:   Write a draft contract and schedule of requirements.

Stage 3 is the actual purchase. POISE exploits the EU restricted procurement procedure which allows the procurer to work with only suitably qualified suppliers at each stage of the process. The steps in stage 3 are:

Step 10:   Issue the EU advert and select capable suppliers.

Step 11:   Issue the statement of need to these suppliers.

Step 12:   Evaluate suppliers' responses and make a first shortlist.

Step 13:   Review the initial shortlist against mandatory requirements and reduce it to a manageable shortlist for tendering.

This stage may also involve issuing the Detailed Statement of Need and obtaining formal responses from suppliers. The tasks and iterative process involved are in many ways similar to preparing the Memorandum of Specification (see below).

Step 14:   Issue the contract framework and discuss this with suppliers, clarifying deliverables, responsibilities and timescales.

Step 15:   Invite tenders.

Step 16: Evaluate suppliers' responses and award contract.
Step 17: Debrief unsuccessful suppliers and publish notice of award.

The fourth stage of POISE is to implementing the contract and realising its benefits. This includes:

Step 18: Implement the contract.
Step 19: Post-acceptance monitoring and benefits realisation analysis.

The cost of the hardware and systems being purchased will determine whether the procurement process must also conform to the European Union General Agreement on Tariffs and Trade Regulations (EU-GATT). The key phases which EU-GATT insist upon are similar to the corresponding POISE steps noted above. EU-GATT demands clearly demonstrable decision points in the procurement process which may be subjected to scrutiny. Good documentation must be maintained to provide an audit trail throughout procurement. Thirteen key phases are involved in a successful procurement under EU-GATT.

Phase I: Initial review of the scope of the procurement: This is a high level review of the scope of the procurement and the agreement of an outline structure for the operational requirement and evaluation model. It is important to confirm the precise boundaries of the procurement and, when identifying an outline operational requirement, to involve all potential users of the system. Successful implementation of the system and the realisation of the benefits expected from it depend on all the users of the system supporting it. This 'ownership' needs to be maintained throughout the procurement. The broad headings to be used within the evaluation model may be identified during this phase.

Phase II: Issue of European Community Journal advertisement: Based on this outline scope for the system, an advertisement will be placed in the *European Community Journal* inviting suppliers to express their interest in the procurement. This advertisement should spell out the precise boundaries of the procurement and the broad evaluation headings to be used to select a first shortlist of suppliers.

Phase III: Developing the detailed operational requirement: The detailed operational requirement is developed on the basis of the outline structure developed in Phase I. It must be so structured that individual suppliers can propose solutions for only part of the required hardware and software. It must also indicate which items suppliers may bid for separately. Now is the time also to begin consulting the potential users about the proposed operational requirements for the system.

Anticipating product trials at phase VII, the operational requirement should ask suppliers to nominate reference sites with a set of clearly defined characteristics such as database size, numbers of tables and individual table sizes, and numbers of concurrent users performing different types of functions. This will identify sites with applications of comparable complexity to the one now being procured.

Phase IV: Finalising and issuing the operational requirement: It is desirable that all potential users of the system to be procured 'own' the operational requirements for it, and essential that there is corporate 'ownership' of the mandatory operational requirements. Failure to comply with the mandatory operation requirements is a sufficient justification, in its own right, to exclude potential suppliers from subsequent phases of the procurement.

Phase V: Developing the evaluation model: For each product identified within the operational requirement a set of evaluation criteria should be developed (and weighted), before the closing date for supplier responses. Between the issue of the operational requirement and this closing date it is desirable to provide interested suppliers with formal opportunity to clarify any uncertainties about the operational requirement and evaluation process. This may take the form of an open day or a series of formal question and answer sessions. It is important to maintain an even-handed approach to all potential suppliers. All questions from suppliers should ideally be dealt with by a single response point and all responses copied to all potential suppliers, eliminating the opportunity for any supplier to question the procurement procedure.

Phase VI: Initial shortlist of potential suppliers: The initial shortlist of suppliers can normally be undertaken in two stages. First, a check must be made that each supplier has complied with the mandatory requirements, set out in the Operational Requirement, to exclude from the full evaluation process any who do not. Subsequently, the responses of each potential supplier will be assessed against the evaluation criteria agreed in Phase V. Suppliers will scrutinise the evaluation because failure at least to reach the shortlist may be seen as damaging their status in the marketplace. Generally, the evaluation process involves scoring the suppliers' responses. To remove bias, various scoring processes have been devised, involving different evaluation team members scoring all suppliers' responses to particular aspects of the requirement, according to their own specific skills and interest, while other members consider a single supplier's response in its entirety. Such approaches are designed to highlight discrepancies in individuals' scoring approaches, allowing these to be investigated.

Phase VII: Review initially-shortlisted suppliers and produce final short-list: Now particular attention may be given to trials of the shortlisted products and evaluating the products' performance at chosen reference sites. Suppliers must be fully informed of both the procedures and environment for any product trials. The evaluation criteria for assessing performance at the reference sites must also be specified. For each reference site visit, a script should be prepared in advance detailing the areas to be covered by questions and by demonstration and made available to suppliers in advance. The Department of Health and RHAs have already prepared standard scripts for

procurements associated with national initiatives such as resource management and HISS. Reference site visits may then be evaluated on the basis of
performance against and compliance with the scripts.

Phase VIII: Development of memoranda of specification: The evaluation
shortlists suppliers. For each supplier, a memorandum of specification will be
prepared. This requires a significant contribution by the potential supplier. It
is important that this process is undertaken in a structured manner and that a
clear timetable is defined at the outset. The objective is to produce a set of
documents which unambiguously define the products and services to be
supplied. With each supplier, a set of formal meetings should take place with
an agenda published for each meeting in advance. Each meeting will cover
one or more areas to be addressed within the memorandum of specification.
Generally, the procuring organisation presents the suppliers with draft
sections of the memorandum of specification. These drafts should clearly
indicate where the supplier is expected to provide a written contribution to
the memorandum of specification. They should be discussed at the meeting
and the suppliers asked to provide their written contributions and any
requests for amendment before the next scheduled meeting.

Failure to comply with this schedule may then lead to the supplier being
excluded from the shortlist. The formality of this process is designed to ensure
that the memoranda of specification are agreed and complete within an
appropriate timescale. This also imposes a discipline on the procuring
organisation to ensure that they enable suppliers to comply with tight
schedules.

Phase IX: Developing and issuing invitations to tender: Taken with the
memoranda of specification, the invitations to tender define unambiguously
the products and services to be supplied. Invitations to tender also specify
terms and conditions for supply. They are issued to shortlisted suppliers who
have signed memoranda of specification. By signing the memorandum of
specification a supplier indicates that they can meet the purchasing organisation's requirements. When evaluating the invitations to tender, the main
issues to be considered are then the prices suppliers have quoted.

Phase X: Developing a tender evaluation model: The selection of suppliers
may be based on the most economically advantageous tender rather than the
least cost tender. The evaluation model must therefore take account of both
the direct costs of the various products and the indirect costs associated with
the use of these products. Within direct costs, the evaluation model must be
capable of digesting potential complexities such as suppliers' alternative
licensing arrangements. These may involve different manufacturers' hardware platforms, different numbers of users on these platforms, the availability of run-time and of development licences. Indirect costs which may be
considered within a tender evaluation model include the training costs with
each supplier's systems and migration costs for the existing applications,
where these are to be ported to hardware being procured. Costs must be

considered over an agreed lifetime for the software product areas to be procured.

Phase XI: Analysing the evaluation of tenders: In this phase it should be possible to bring together all aspects of the cost of each product, or product set, and to establish any added value of combinations which might occur.

Phase XII: Recommendations for award of contracts: A fully documented report covering all aspects of the procurement must be developed at this phase. Detailed debriefing notes should be produced to debrief unsuccessful suppliers in a consistent fashion. It is important that the report clearly identifies unsuccessful suppliers' shortcomings in relationship to the evaluation criteria and models used when shortlisting and at final selection.

Phase XIII: Post-contractual negotiations: Inevitably a large procurement will result in significant post-contractual negotiations with the preferred suppliers before the final contractual matters are settled.

There is a danger that the procurement process may become a mechanistic series of steps in which you lose sight of the real purpose of procurement. Manuel argues that:

> the choice of what type of system to buy and from whom to buy it is not one that can be made rationally . . . ultimately it is the artistic side of the process that decides success. (Manuel 1991: 28)

In managing this artistic part of the process internally one has to decide who should be involved and how to ensure that the process and the developing needs of the organisation in the fast changing NHS are kept together, and how to face the critical task of implementation. Devolution of procurement to individual providers or purchasing bodies gives an opportunity to ensure that local requirements are met and that staff within the organisation feel committed to or have a sense of ownership of the system. There is also the danger, however, that user requirements become practically unachievable resulting in strange modifications to packages that run perfectly well elsewhere, pushing up costs dramatically. Successful procurement and implementation of information systems requires a good working partnership between purchaser and supplier. Both parties must feel happy, not just with the deal struck but that expectations, responsibilities, deadlines and resources are clear. This places the responsibility on both purchaser and potential supplier to be open, honest and fair, and on the purchaser to be clear and firm about their needs and expectations of the product and the service. However, a key ingredient of a successful partnership is that the organisations – and that means the people who work for them – get on together. The rules for managing relations with external consultancies are similar, much as in other areas of management.

The generalist manager brings to the IT procurement process the artistry of management. To be effective in doing that she needs to be able to apply general management skills to information systems procurement but she also needs to understand what it is that the organisation is trying to procure. Manuel suggests that 'Knowing about the suppliers and technology is useful. Knowing your own organisation is essential' (Manuel 1991: 28). It is the effective application of that knowledge to the needs of the organisation that ensures success.

Chapter 12

THE FUTURE OF
UK HEALTH INFORMATICS

Rod Sheaff

Determining the development agenda

UK health system reforms suggest research, development and policy agendas for health service information systems. What kinds of information systems are relevant to a health system depends upon four aspects of the whole health system. Substantive health policy determines what indicators, monitoring variables, data sets, definitions and standards must be used for reporting to central bodies. The health system structure (in effect, its property relations (Enthoven 1991; Maynard 1991)) determines whether its constituent organisations prioritise commercial or health gain objectives, and what networking is required between them. It also determines their internal organisation; how decentralised they are, how much discretion individual managers have and what their practical interests are. All this determines the content and purposes of information systems at local, organisational level. A health system's structure lastly determines how open it is to external technological and organisational influences on its working practices and information systems.

Technical and commercial developments in other sectors, and the commercial ambitions of IT and information system suppliers, have strongly influenced the information systems now on offer to healthcare organisations. So there is no guarantee that the available technology matches the objectives of the healthcare organisation. Two kinds of mismatch occur. One is technical underdevelopment, given the organisational and health system imperatives; its converse is organisational incapacity to exploit technical possibilities.

Technical underdevelopment occurs when information systems do not adequately serve the objectives of the health system or its constituent organisations, failing to produce the kind, quantity or distribution of information necessary to enable managers and organisations to meet these objectives. To identify areas of technical underdevelopment one therefore takes the health system structure and objectives as given. One then compares the information systems such a health system implicitly requires with its actual information systems. The differences indicate priorities for technical health service information system research and development.

Conversely, organisational underdevelopment can be defined as the ways in which the existing health system structure and objectives prevent full use of the information-producing capabilities of existing or foreseeable information systems or technologies for purposes of health gain. Previous chapters identified many areas of technical underdevelopment in NHS information systems. This chapter offers some technical development proposals to address them. For the immediate future UK health policy seems relatively stable; but since, in the longer term, there may be opportunity to reform the reforms, this chapter also considers some areas of organisational under-development.

Technical development of information systems

Since the NHS reforms have parallels in other countries (see Chapter 1), so will some of the information consequences. One parallel is the differentiation of two main types of health organisations: those planning and financing the system; and those directly providing services. Different organisational objectives imply different information system requirements (see Chapter 1). So the respects in which their existing information systems are technically underdeveloped may differ for different types of health service organisation. In most health systems (including Britain's) different health organisations pursue different mixtures of health gain, political and commercial objectives. Health gain and political objectives dominate the purchasing level of the NHS, commercial objectives increasingly dominating at trust level.

Insofar as they are not simply intrinsic to any health system, NHS health gain objectives are partly a residue of 1976 planning systems and RAWP (Resource Allocation Working Party) (indeed of the postwar settlement of health policy), partly a result of the public health renaissance for which the WHO deserves much credit. Even private, for-profit healthcare providers pursue health gain objectives insofar as there are commercial imperatives for doing so (for example in risk management, in the US case). NHS health gain objectives currently emphasise service quality, not only the administrative matters covered by the *Patient's Charter* but also the clinical outcome of healthcare, of which clinical audit is seen as the main guarantor. *Health of the Nation* adds demands for more effective needs assessment, for more coordination of the health and non-health sectors system, and for more active health promotion, especially in the six areas prioritised in that document. Social and community care, has among others, both a preventive and a therapeutic rationale (Department of Health 1992).

What technical development NHS purchaser information systems require can be identified by comparing the information already available to purchasers with the information profile their new roles actually demand. Chapter 3 dealt with this from the DHA standpoint and Chapter 4 from that of GP (including fundholder) and FHSA information systems. Chapter 2 outlined the current state of NHS information strategy. In summary, they suggest the main purchaser information system developments which remain outstanding, will then be to:

1 Unify the healthcare purchasing information systems of DHAs with those of other DHAs and FHSAs, to exploit economies of scale, to increase the range of providers which each purchasing organisation faces locally and to simplify coordination with local authority social services. If integrated purchasing and integrated information systems have much to recommend them the obvious conclusion is that integrated purchasing organisations, for health and social services, are desirable too.
2 Develop data collection systems to enable purchasers to produce pertinent, comprehensive health profiles. Patient data from GPs is an obvious source to exploit.
3 Research further the factors influencing health status, quantify how far healthcare can influence these factors and how far intersectoral action can.
4 Considerably strengthen information systems for managing public health and health promotion.
5 Extend the SID work on best practice protocols, especially to health promotion and long-stay social care (or initiate similar work); and develop benchmarking to cover all current types of health service and those under evaluation and piloting.
6 Develop, standardise and implement health status (and outcome) indicators.
7 Develop iso-outcome besides iso-resource case mix groupers.
8 Revise the so-called efficiency indicators on the above basis.
9 Refine the decision rules that purchaser information systems will have to operate by, using qualitative applied research in decision theory and healthcare ethics.

Scope for technical development in the information systems of GPs and trusts, long-term care and health promoters can also be identified by comparing the demands posed by the reformed health system with the state of their current information systems. An internal market gives NHS trusts expressly commercial objectives. In the late 1990s this necessitates developing marketing information systems and information systems for contract management in particular. As the internal market develops, what information will be necessary to manage a trust's contracts will depend on the nature of its marketing activity.

A starting-point is a market analysis showing what purchasers there are, purchaser market segments (HAs, GPFHs, ECRs, private patients), and effective demand for each service in cash, referral, service contract and ECR terms. Analysing these flows by source and destination shows how much work each purchaser sends to the trust and how much to competitors. Workflows to other providers catering for the same patient groups as a trust indicate who its actual competitors; flows of local patients to more distant providers suggest that the latter offer benefits outwieghing the inconvenience. Comparing total demand with purchasers' actual utilisation of the trust shows potential new work. Comparing total purchaser demand with the total capacity of all local providers gives a first indication of a trust's bargaining power in the local market. Financial or contracting information systems, and the PAS, is the obvious source of at least the utilisation data for this analysis. Data for the total demand side will have to come from DHAs, FHSAs or even RHAs (especially where there are large cross-boundary flows). It is especially important to know why these flows occur; what purchasers, GPs and users see as the trust's main strengths and weakness compared with alternative providers. This requires routine surveying of DHAs (or consortia), GPFHs, GPs and prospective patients.

A situation analysis shows how these factors are likely to change. One common form is a PEST (Political, Economic, Social, Technical) analysis of the:

1 Political climate, such as new policy on public access to information, the *Patients Charter* and new rules for costing and pricing (see below).
2 Social factors influencing patient flows and case-mix, such as demographic and epidemiological changes (e.g. more 'old elderly' patients), changes in occupational patterns and unemployment, lifestyles and health behaviours (e.g. declines in smoking except among young working-class women, later childbearing among professional women).
3 Substitutes for existing services, whether new technologies (e.g. PET scanning, genotyping), new models of care (e.g. community care replacing long-stay hospitals, consultants outpatient clinics at fundholders' practices instead of hospital) or new providers.

Standard methods are available for analysing market, demographic and social data (e.g. ACORN, JICNARS; see Chisnall 1991; Chapter 6) which NHS trusts could adopt. Where there is a significant private health sector, publications such as Laing's *Review of Private Healthcare* (Laing, annually) indicate private providers' main activities, hence what selling points might be attractive to private healthcare purchasers.

Market analyses demand both re-analyses of existing data (using the existing information systems) and *ad hoc* market research which consolidates by repetition into a marketing information system of its own (Sheaff 1991a). Deciding the trust's marketing mix requires information on service quality, price and promotion. Chapter 6 outlined what information systems trusts might require for managing service quality.

Trust information systems will have to support a marketing decision on what pricing strategy to adopt (supposing trusts are allowed more latitude in future), and contract management decisions on how to ensure long-run price sustainability and how to relate prices to case mix. At present, RHAs publish competitors' pricing in the annual, fixed tariffs but in the future more price flexibility may be allowed, especially, *Working For Patients* suggested, in respect of pricing marginal spare capacity (Department of Health 1989a: 35). In pricing service contracts the two main considerations are competitors' pricing and the trust's own costs. While prices are based directly on costs (NHSME 1990, 1992) they can be calculated simply by adding the permitted 6 per cent 'surplus' (i.e. profit) to costs and comparing the result with competitors' prices. Trust information systems must therefore calculate these costs and model how they respond to variations in throughput, occupancy, length of stay etc. The simplest way is in terms of variable, semi-variable and fixed costs per patient for each service contract (Babson 1973: 11). Even in this simple a pricing system, trust negotiators need to know the sensitivity of total costs to different apportionment assumptions in terms of cash and patient flows for the best, worst and likeliest cases. This shows the trust's negotiator what bargaining concessions he or she can safely offer (e.g. discounts for bulk, off-peak, marginal contracts) (one illustration is in Sheaff 1991: 106). Software already exists in the USA to enable providers to 'optimise' the coding of individual patients to maximise payments from purchasers (Newman and Jenkins 1991: 51). In the longer term NHS trusts might acquire an incentive to copy this, although that would be a clear instance of a perverse incentive in the development of information systems.

Purchasers might reasonably seek reassurance from the trust's negotiators that their trust can sustain the prices it offers through the contract period and, for the present, that it has priced on the centrally prescribed basis (see above). All costings have to be updated periodically as methods of care and input costs change but this task is readily automated. If NHS pricing rules relax in future, trusts will require more flexible modelling of the relations between prices, workload, income, costs and profits, again for pricing and negotiating purposes. As Chapter 9 explains, this demands case mix systems that can separately calculate the effects of case mix changes upon costs and upon income. In these ways, costing information supports a trust's marketing.

Managing cost-and-volume contracts requires either an information system that can place each referral in a standard broad charging category; or one which assembles individual patient bills from a set of charges for items of service (per bed-day, theatre sessions, drug use, etc.) much as private hospitals do, except that NHS trusts would presumably also have to apportion and charge medical staff costs. The NHSME's generic case mix system specification (Bullas 1989: 13) recommends costing on the basis of standard event costs, updated monthly (or preferably annually) to avoid recording cost data in every patient record. Diseconomies of scale set in when one tries to increase the accuracy of health service costings, because of the increased size and complexity of the financial information systems. These diseconomies can be minimised by 'bundling' services to produce the largest service contracts that purchasers will accept: where possible, block or cost-and-volume contracts with HAs and small block contracts with GP fundholders (e.g. for 20 or 40 patients) for routine procedures such as cataract extraction. Practically it is more important to be able to calculate the approximate sizes of a trust's main cost drivers (e.g. ICU stays, unplanned readmissions) than the last detail of relatively insignificant costs. Ideally, trust information systems would be able to calculate individual patient costings and event costings, but exceptionally not routinely, to identify and analyse outlier high cost or high risk cases (e.g. small neonates, HIV, multiple trauma/ICU patients) and, periodically, causes of variance of individual patient costs (Benson 1991: 56–7). Some individual pricing of ECRs may be inescapable.

Prompt and complete billing, to sustain a trust's cash flow, is an obvious area for automation using computerised contract management information systems. Early experience of the internal market, especially in London, has demonstrated how urgent it is for trusts to be able quickly to monitor completed workload against service contract targets. With simple block contracts a trust's PAS need only identify each patient's DHA or GP fundholder and speciality, distinguish GPFH cases costing over £5000 per annum and detect, cost and bill ECRs. Whatever form of contract is used, a trust's billing system would generate data quantifying progress towards exhausting the service contract (a sensitive issue in 1993) and income still due, attributing these to the appropriate external purchaser and the relevant internal department or directorate budgets. All these would be important data for the next round of market analysis (see above).

One way a THIS (see Chapter 1) can be used is to transmit routine monitoring data on-line to purchasers. Some private UK healthcare purchasers make compatability between information systems in the (private) hospitals they use and their own information systems a condition of using that hospital. NHS purchasers might do likewise and NHSME expects all new trust information systems to satisfy its *Common Basic Specification* (Bullas 1989), although in 1993 not above 100 NHS trusts possessed any form of HISS (Fairey 1993). Conversely, it would be reasonable for trusts to include these costs in the corresponding service prices. On US experience, hospitals could be networked to GPs through EDI (Benson 1991: 43; see Chapter 1) for routine referrals, discharges, billing and clinical data transfer between GP and hospital. Proposed as long ago as 1916, standardised health records are the logical culmination of data standardisation. They would allow automated clinical data transfer throughout the NHS. Many US hospitals sub-contract this routine administration to specialist firms who thereby amass enormous databases, valuable both for management and research purposes (McCord 1993).

Besides the points discussed in Chapter 4, fundholding gives GPs an incentive to introduce IT-based substitutions for secondary care, such as telemedicine consultation with hospital doctors (Benson 1991: 8), expert databases (cf. WHO 1988: 55–6) and telediagnostics. In principle, all GPs could use the resulting technology. It has been suggested that videotex systems could be developed to provide them with occupational health updates and clinical information on conditions which they rarely see. All these are rich areas for technical research and development.

Comparing these requirements with the information systems which Chapters 4, 5, 6 and 11 mention reveals some striking contrasts.

For market analysis, the position is simple: virtually no information systems exist, even manual ones, although there has been one attempt to launch a subscriber database on NHS purchasers' purchasing patterns. The EU-funded MEMPHIS (Measuring and Economic Modelling of the Performance of Healthcare through Information Systems) project addresses some economic aspects of PEST analysis (Fisher and Kitson 1993).

Trusts' market research mainly takes the form of surveys of patients and GPs (especially fundholders) but little up-to-date evidence is publicly available to quantify the extent or summarise results. In 1986, Guttman and Annandale had already recorded 105 consumer relations training projects in the NHS, but only 40 respondents mentioned market research. It is easier to find evidence that quality management activities occur in NHS trusts than evidence of any actual impact on service quality or outcome. Standard-setting projects under the national TQM initiatives and some Regional projects (e.g. in Trent RHA) engendered *ad-hoc* local information systems for service quality management. Some of these can report activity levels against standards but few if any are sophisticated enough to support statistical process control. Clinical research apart, neither the quality indicators nor the corresponding data are practically available to NHS managers. The proposed national database of quality indicators may palliate the first difficulty. Although work continues (e.g. Richards 1993: 211–42; Ifeachor 1993) clinical decision support systems remain experimental. While they are NHS-wide comparative data, the Körner data-sets (NHSME 1991a) largely match professional 'data fiefdoms' and few indicate service quality. English

Resource Management case mix systems did adopt a 'product line' approach through the requirement to construct normal care profiles (Benson 1991: 27) and work constructing care profiles did begin (e.g. NHSME 1991b). The idea of using care profiles reportedly gained some clinical acceptance in the RMI pilot sites (Health Economics Research Group 1991: 10). How this work will be developed remains unclear in 1994.

Pricing and costing information systems at least function in NHS trusts; but erratically. A study of one NHS Region in 1992 reported prices for skin biopsies ranging from £91 to £1165, and prices for treatments of varicosity from £287 to £1278 (Northern RHA 1994). Such divergences are not confined to one region. Partly they reflect different clinical practices (especially lengths of stay) but also inconsistencies, different methods, different assumptions and straightforward mistakes in costing. Costing data inherited from the pre-reform NHS focused on events (patient ambulance journey, weighted patient day, etc.) not episodes of care (CIPFA 1987) and were analysed geographically and by speciality, not by provider. The Resource Management projects (see Packwood *et al.* 1991) seem to have been abandoned. The Financial Information Project may ultimately develop into a patient-based financial system but at present (1994) assembles mainly input costs at a fairly gross level (e.g. the annual cost of a health visitor) without attributing them to patient episodes or events. Proprietary costing and case mix systems are being developed but even the apparent market leader's (ATT-ISTEL) generates only a narrow range of direct costs (drugs, consumables, etc.) on a patient-episode basis. Case-mix systems are being developed (see Chapters 3, 5 and 9) but before a trust can use even these its THIS must first supply the necessary data. Chapter 2 outlined NHS strategy for developing THISs through the HISS project. Chapter 7 indicated some of the difficulties in implementing NHS trust information systems in general.

Community Information System for Purchasers (CISP) is to be constructed similarly. Following pilot projects in Devon and Dorset in 1988 IMG proposed the automation of GP-FHSA links handling registration and service fee claims using EDI (see Chapter 1). Twelve pilot projects were due for completion during 1993. Most existing GP information systems automate the registers and financial systems. In Oxford and Northampton EDI transmission between GPs and hospitals of pathology test requests, test results and waiting list information is being piloted (Daniels *et al.* 1993). Five DHAs and an RHA are running pilot schemes provide GPs with on-line information on hospital waiting times. All this is part of a wider IMG strategy for NHS-wide networking (see Chapter 2). IMG has decided that future developments will focus on collecting and networking GP data on morbidity and mortality of individual patients and priority target groups, and the management of GPs' contracts. Read codes will be used to codify the clinical data.

Call and recall systems, practice list maintenance, clinic scheduling and billing FHSAs are obvious areas for automating routine GP administration. To achieve the 100 per cent level (or nearly) FHSAs might consider giving GPs information systems in return for access to some of the resulting data, as drugs firms have (Benson 1991: 42). Chapter 4 indicated that in these areas, GP systems are already comparatively widespread and well developed. By analogy with the levels of computerisation achieved in GP pharmacies it is already realistic to envisage a target of nearly 100 per cent of general practices having at least partly computerised administration (cf. Benson 1991: 2). The System Accreditation Project for Primary Healthcare Information require-ments and Evaluations (SAPPHIRE) is producing software for testing proprietary GP information systems against a minimum system specification. GPs who purchase information systems will only be reimbursed if their system satisfies this specification.

Supposing the aforementioned developmental projects continue, all this suggests the following main directions for technical development of provider information systems. Although they have IT implications their solutions depend much more on articulating exactly what information the new systems ought to produce, why and for whom:

1 Creating systems for trusts' market analyses including the qualitative aspects, regular market research and market databases.
2 Developing outcome and health status indicators and the corresponding data collection systems to the point where statistical process control of clinical quality is possible. Hence:
3 A degree of standardisation of medical records (see Chapter 8), including standard health indicators, data fields and definitions, and:
4 Developing clinical protocols and clinical decision support systems, and:
5 Starting work on iso-outcome case mix systems.
6 Innovating IT-based means for GP care to replace hospital-based diagnosis and treatment (telediagnosis, etc).
7 Continued development of trust costing systems, especially their modelling capacity, with emphasis on producing valid approximations of service costs.
8 Continued development of iso-resource case mix systems.
9 Implementation studies to identify the practical means of realising the potential benefits of the new information systems.

To select which indicators are used for monitoring healthworkers' performance (and so for determining their rewards, whether in terms of cash, career or professional credibility) is to select which outcomes these health-workers have an incentive to demonstrate they have achieved. (Reciprocally the incentives give the healthworkers reason to maximise collection of the corresponding data; for example an important incentive for automating the routine administration of general practices has been to demonstrate target achievement for payment purposes (Benson 1991: 43; and see Chapter 4).)

The character of these indicators and information systems is therefore the legitimate concern not purely of managers, informaticians and doctors but of policy makers and the general public.

Information and health policy

When health services are reformed technical development of information systems almost inevitably follows. Conversely, changes in health policy and health system structure become necessary when health system organisation frustrates the possibilities for health gain which new information systems and technologies offer. Although the NHS reform is still being implemented and government's views about what kind of internal market to create are vague, some organisational obstacles to exploiting health information systems can be anticipated from other economic sectors' and other health systems' experiences. Looking beyond the NHS's immediate information strategy (see Chapter 2), these organisational problems suggest priorities both for NHS informatic research, development, and information policy; and for health policy itself.

Because competing providers have to do their business planning, financial planning, consumer and market research independently (Rea 1993 elaborates) the necessary information systems have to replicated in each. It might be argued (although *Working for Patients* does not) that this replication creates a 'requisite variety' of technical innovations in methods for collecting, analysing and presenting information. Internal markets also encourage providers to specialise in specific market niches, hence develop correspondingly specialised provider information systems.

'Requisite' as variety in information systems may be for encouraging innovation, its effects in making common data sets, standards, definitions and analyses, hardware protocols and specifications, data networking, aggregation and comparison difficult to establish are far from requisite. Fragmentation of the NHS into an internal market threatens the availability, validity and completeness of information about health service efficacy and management. Before the reforms DHAs implemented (with varying degrees of success) distict-wide patient record systems and call and recall systems, and could easily produce district-wide service profiles. To suggest that this unusual – if seldom noticed – strength of the pre-reform NHS might be at risk from technical diversification is no idle fear, remembering the incompatible designs of patient-held smart cards (even of floppy disc sizes and formats) advanced in the 1980s. Replicating systems also replicates administrative costs. Such problems already occur even within NHS trusts. Between trusts, it makes the purchasers' job of comparing healthcare providers unnecessarily difficult. Community care policy presents these difficulties in especially acute form because it anticipates provision of care by diverse suppliers: NHS trusts, local authority social services, voluntary bodies, charities, and commercial providers (Department of Health 1988: 5–6, 15–20, 25–6). The problem becomes bigger as an EU-wide market for healthcare begins to materialise in a few services; Danish patients travel to Spain, and Italians to Russia for cold ophthalmic surgery; southern English DHAs have already considered buying cold surgery in northern France. Firms from the mainland are already tendering for ancillary services for NHS Trusts; there seems little reason for information services to escape this process (for a review of EU policy on healthcare, see Altenstetter (1991)).

Before the reforms NHS providers usually shared data and information openly and without charge, in contrast to private health firms. No longer; property rights in information and knowledge are a corollary of an internal market system (and being created *de facto* irrespective of official recognition). There are reports that NHS information itself is becoming a commodity (e.g. *The Guardian* 31 July 1991). Since the late 1980s NHS units have sold income generation ideas to each other and data to pharmaceutical and other businesses. It is reasonable to assume that competition impedes dissemination of information, and of knowledge of good management practice. In markets information on commodity costs and quality becomes a selling tool. A monopoly of it gives bargaining advantage. At best this creates incentives for provider secrecy ('commercial confidentiality'), at worst it presents patients, the public and purchasers with partial, misleading or false data. NHS policy documents expressly require purchasers to respect providers' commercial confidentiality and tacitly recognise that unscrupulous providers have an incentive to mislead (NHSME 1993b).

A policy dilemma is therefore whether to let competition promote variety and rapid innovation in information systems but risk losing trustworthy NHS-wide data and reducing the manageability of the internal market; or to do the opposite.

Although governments had political incentives to offer partial or misleading data to the public long before the NHS reforms, controversies over health policy have reinforced them. One motive for the reforms appears to have been to distance government from unpopular decisions about levels of NHS funding, indeed to discourage NHS managers from addressing the question at all (cf. Department of Health 1988: iii–ix; Bottomley 1993), and from the consequent 'rationing' decisions. However government also seeks evidence of health policy 'success'. A consequence has been adjusting information systems to obfuscate politically sensitive data. One example is the redefinition and trimming of hospital waiting lists and times just before the 1992 election (Mullen 1992); another is redefining NHS hospital activity in terms of 'completed consultant episodes' instead of completed treatment plans, inflating patient numbers by some millions (Seng *et al.* 1993; McKee 1993). Other information flows, for instance on *Patient's Charter* and the purchaser efficiency index are created specifically for monitoring implementation of political initiatives. Governments have also tried to conceal information on health promotion and intersectoral action. The Black Report was first published as 200 photocopies of typescript on a bank holiday weekend (DHSS 1980). The Smee Report appeared only because ministers had promised Parliament, and then without the opening summary stating that tobacco advertising does somewhat increase the incidence of smoking (Smee 1992).

Yet the reforms are also compelling NHS purchasers to consider explicitly whether local health services produce as much health gain as budgets allow and minimise iatrogenesis. At trust and directorate level, government looks to clinical audit to guarantee this. Reliance on clinical audit has the advantage of taking these questions of health gain and iatrogenesis to the heart of health care. Its disadvantage is that the clinical audit remains predominantly under professional control, with the risk of restricting the availability of information about the outcomes and quality of care on such grounds as confidentiality and clinical autonomy. The relation between clinicians and managers which makes this restriction possible stems from the settlement between government and the medical profession when the NHS was founded.

Markets intrinsically demand parallel information systems, one dealing with the real and one with the financial aspects of health care; a second duplication of information systems. Its opportunity cost is the foregone opportunities to develop information systems dealing with the 'real side' of healthcare; health gain. Commercialised information systems naturally focus on finance and in developing NHS information systems UK governments have given earlier and higher priority to developing financial information systems (The Resource Management Initiative (RMI) and its successors) than to developing outcome indicators or comparative clinical evaluations of the effectiveness of different patterns of care. Because the choice of monitoring indicator is tantamount to the choice of incentives for NHS providers there are obviously further, non-informational dangers in implementing NHS information systems which monitor providers more by activity levels and financial results than health gain.

The closer to individual patient and procedure level pricing and costing is taken, the bigger the opportunity cost embodied in financial information and administration (billing, payment etc.) systems. The danger is, that the (often *ad hoc*) information systems already created for resource management and to handle ECRs are the top of a 'slippery slope' at the bottom of which lie individualised case-cost or procedure-cost systems on the US model. This danger exists on the purchaser side of the internal market too. If it led in this direction, the proposed Guernsey experiment in compulsory private health insurance would be another retrograde move in terms of developing cheap, outcome-orientated health information systems. Although figures are contested it has been argued that approximately $13 billion of the cost of the US health system can be attributed to its transaction costs (Brandon et al. 1991).

(Beveridge found transaction costs ranging from 6 per cent to 10 per cent in the pre-NHS British health system (Beveridge 1942: 73,160).) A warning sign is the rise in managerial staffing and costs during the NHS reforms (*The Guardian* 7 January 1993). Although this increase has other causes besides new financial information systems it is a retrograde outcome of reforms whose stated aims include reducing bureaucracy and diverting the savings to patient care (Bottomley 1993).

Managing the internal market necessitates strong, active NHS purchasers. Partly this depends upon purchasers having strong information systems (see Chapter 3), partly on reducing their organisational fragmentation. The proposed reform of HAs (Department of Health 1993d) goes some way to meet these problems although the inchoate proposals for local government reform still complicate matters. Coterminosity with local authorities would facilitate joint planning purposes (especially community care and community health services), data sharing and comparison.

One set of policy responses to these problems lies in the areas of intellectual property rights in information and innovation.

The obvious response to the risks of commercial and governmental concealment and falsification of information requires statutory, even constitutional reform. An open information policy would place the onus of argument on those who would restrict access to NHS managerial information and to information on health and health policy at governmental level. A corollary is the civil right for NHS staff to publish health information (except information on individual patients) without penalty, when publication is bona fide, even though the information might be politically controversial or embarrass managers, government or business. Since the NHS is intended to provide more or less comprehensive health care, it would appear that such a policy should extend not only to NHS hospitals but to general practices, social care organisations, preventive and intersectoral activity, and private sector providers. One way to implement the policy would be to make access to information a condition for receiving NHS money. Chapter 3 notes what managerial information some US purchasers publish to help consumers evaluate alternative healthcare providers and health services planning. It can be argued that summary clinical audit results ought to be included in an open information policy, although Watkins' (1987: 18f,74,167f) remarks suggest that the UK medical profession is unlikely to welcome this spontaneously. A presumption of access to documents would incidentally discourage parallel, private 'unofficial' information and records systems (cf. Chapter 8).

Prima facie there are sound arguments for exempting non-anonymised personal health records and staff records from an open information policy. In respect of commercial confidentiality, the dilemma mentioned above justifies only a qualified exemption.

A palliative response is to regulate that all NHS bodies supply purchasing and regulatory bodies with common minimum sets of data, constructed by using NHS-wide, or preferably EU-wide, data codes, standards and definitions for health information. EU health information policy is addressing EU-wide data standards, developing EMEDI as the European standard for medical electronic data interchange, and proposing training strategies on health informatics (Council of Europe 1991). *EC Decision 87/95/EEC* of 1989 already requires procurers of all public sector information systems to order only systems meeting OSI (Open Systems Interconnection) standards (Benson 1991: 82–4,90). Europe-wide work is under way to standardise registration and identification of coding schemes for EDI in healthcare but not yet to standardise codes themselves (Markwell 1993), as are a pilot scheme ('MEDICINE') on medical data interchange between EU countries and work on the architecture of a European health record.

Necessary as this is it does little to stimulate or harness innovations in healthcare informatics themselves. The variety-versus-standardisation dilemma arises because in markets the normal way of 'rewarding' organisations which innovate profitable new information systems or technologies is that the innovator has intellectual property in the innovation. This either gives competitive advantage or a practical monopoly in the innovation. The consequent rewards depend on excluding competitors from using the innovation except on the innovator's terms, or at all. The solution to this dilemma must lie in finding ways to reward such innovations without limiting their dissemination. One way would be, for NHSME to encourage diversity during the innovation stage of the lifecycle of new information systems but stipulate that intellectual property rights in information systems or technologies developed by NHS bodies pass automatically to them for free NHS-wide dissemination, in return for a mandatory but generous reward to the innovator.

To ensure that internal market incentives reward the achievement of health gain, in both curative and health promotion services, rather than the sale of curative health services, requires a policy of making outcome indicators the main medium of monitoring, hence incentivising, providers. Iso-outcome case mix systems are required if purchasers are to compare providers (making them compete) on a basis of achieved health gain standardised for case mix. This would also advance the development of benchmarking current best practice on a real health gain basis, taking benchmarking down to the level of clinical practice. The culmination of such a policy would be a contract pricing system based on the proportion of achievable health gain actually achieved, not on service-event pricing, and this at care-group rather than at individual patient level. The first experiment in outcome pricing is due to begin in 1994.

So critical is information to this, and to purchasers' attempts to manage the internal market in general, that information considerations should strongly influence policy on the structure of the purchasing side of the internal market. Purchaser information costs – of expert staff besides hardware and software – show economies of scale. At 1994 UK prices it costs roughly £2 million annually to run a purchaser organisation with a public health, finance, planning and general management function. This cost varies little for population sizes of 200 000 or 2 million; and information quality tends to be higher with the larger population because analyses, projections and modelling become more accurate. For managing the internal market there are obvious advantages in networking, even integrating, the information systems of the corresponding FHSAs, health and local authorities. These are prima facie reasons for integrating health and social services purchasing organisations on the scale of the pre–1982 Area Health Authorities or (in local government terms), of the counties. As near-monopsonies in local internal markets purchasers this size would have a strong bargaining position in the face of service providers. This proposal leaves open the questions whether the purchase of secondary health service is better left to fundholders and whether intersectoral activity (with its heavy reliance on publicising health and epidemiological information) should be contracted to specialist providers or undertaken on a directly managed basis by the purchasing organisations themselves.

A central health policy problem is, how to steer the internal market reforms in the UK (and elsewhere) towards a health system structure that creates incentives for health organisations to define, monitor, and reward health gain; and to withstand pressures to subordinate this to public expenditure containment, electoralism or healthcare commercialisation for its own sake. The design and outputs of health information systems can contribute. Not the least task of those who theorise, design and operate health service information systems is to ensure that they do.

REFERENCES

Abbott, B. (1986). 'The problem of IT in the NHS', *Information and Public Policy*, **xv** pp. 1–5, 1, Winter.

Abbott, W. (ed.) (1993). *Information Technology in Healthcare. A Handbook.* Harlow, Kluwer and Institute of Health Services Management.

Ackoff, P.L. (1976). 'Management Misinformation Systems' in Davis, G. and Everest, M.G.C. (eds) *Readings in Management Information Systems.* Maidenhead, McGraw-Hill.

Aldridge, S.J., Cronin, E. and Wastell, D. (1988) 'A socio-technical approach to healthcare systems' in Richards (1988) pp. 171–75.

Aldridge, S.J. and Walker, H. (1991). 'Resource management and medical records', *The Journal for Health Care Information and Medical Records*, **xxxii**, 4, November, 2–4.

Allison, D.J. and Martin, N. (1993). 'PACS: what the user wants', in Richards (1993) pp. 347–55.

AMRO (Association of Health Care Information and Medical Records Officers) (1985). *Handbook for Quality Control in Medical Records.* London, AMRO and MDU.

Anderson, J.G., Jay, S.J., Schweer, H. and Anderson, M.M. (1986). 'Why doctors don't use computers: some empirical findings', *Journal of the Royal Society of Medicine*, **lxxix**, March, 142–4.

Anon (1991). *The Read Codes.* Loughborough, Computer Aided Medical Systems Limited.

Anon (1991–2). *Yorkshire Region. Read Code Evaluation Study* Warrington, Computer Services Ltd and HSMU.

Anon (1992). 'Experten von Koalition und SPD einig uber Eckwerte fur die Gesundheitsreform', *Suddeutscher Zeitung*, 5 October 1992.

Ashmore, M., Mulkay, M. and Pinch, T. (1989). *Health and Efficiency: A Sociology of Economics.* Buckingham, Open University Press.

Ashworth, C. and Woodland, M. (1990). *SSADM. A Practical Approach*. Maidenhead, McGraw-Hill.

Atkinson, C.J. (1992). *The Information Function in Health Care Organisations* Manchester, HSMU.

Atkinson, P. (1981). *The Clinical Experience. The Construction and Reconstruction of Medical Reality*. Gower, Farnborough.

Audit Commission (1990). *A Short Cut to Better Services*. London, HMSO.

Audit Commission (1992). *Report and Accounts, year ended 31 March 1992*, London, HMSO.

Audit Commission (1993). *Their Health, Your Business: The New Role of the District Health Authority*. London, HMSO.

Australian Council on Hospital Standards (annually). *The Accreditation Guide – Standards for Australian Health Care Facilities*. Sydney, Australian Council for Hospital Standards.

Avison, D.E. and Fitzgerald, G. (1988). *Information Systems Development. Methodologies, Techniques and Tools*. Oxford, Blackwell.

Babson, J.H. (1973). *Disease Costing*. Manchester, Manchester University Press.

Baird, R. (1992). 'Running Out of Steam', *Health Services Journal*, 11 June 1992, pp. 26–7.

Ball, M.J., Douglas, J.V., O'Desky, R.I. and Albright, J.W. (eds) (1991). Healthcare Information Management Systems – A Practical Guide. New York, Springer-Verlag.

Bardsley, M., Coles, J. and Jenkins, L. (eds) (1987). *DRGs and Health Care*. London, King's Fund.

Benefits Realisation Advisory Group (1994). *Guidance on Benefits Realisation*. Cardiff, Welsh Office.

Benson, T. (1991). *Medical Informatics*. Harlow, Longman.

Beveridge, W. (1942). *Social Insurance and Allied Services*, in the Beveridge Report. London, HMSO.

Blackler, F. and Brown, C. (1986) 'Alternative models to guide the design and introduction of the new information technologies into work organisations', *Journal of Occupational Psychology*, lix, 287–313.

Bock, F.M. (1982). 'Considering human factors in the initial analysis and design of a medical computer system', *Journal of Medical Systems*, vi, 61–8.

Boissier de Sauvages de Lacroix, F. (1768). *Nosologia Methodica Systens Morborum Classus Juxta Sidenhami Mentum et Botanicorum Ordinem*. Naples: Manfredius.

Boss, R. (1989). *Organisational Development in Healthcare*. Reading, Mass., Addison Wesley.

Bostrum, R.P. and Heinen, J.S. (1977). 'MIS problems and failures: a socio-technical perspective', *MIS Quarterly*, xvi, 17–32.

Bottomley, V. (1992). Speech to 1992 NAHA conference; reported in Brindle, D. 'Make better use of funds NHS warned', *The Guardian*, 25 September 1992, p. 5.

Bottomley, V. (1993). Speech to 1993 NAHAT conference; reported in *The Health Summary*, x, 2 February 1993, 1.

Bourn, A. (1987). 'Fighting truth decay in the NHS', *Accountancy*, September. xix, 17–20.

Bourn, M. and Ezzamel, M. (1986a). 'Costing and Budgeting in the National Health Service', *Financial Accountability and Management*, ii, 1, Spring, 53–71.

Bourn, M. and Ezzamel, M. (1986b). 'Organisational culture in Hospitals in the National Health Service', *Financial Accountability and Management*, ii, 3, 203–25.

Bowling, A. (1991). *Measuring Health. A Review of Quality of Life Measurement Scales*. Buckingham, Open University Press.

Bradley, P. (1993). 'Towards holistic audit', *Journal of Informatics in Primary Care*, January, 3–6.

Brandon, R.M., Podhorzer, M. and Pollak, T.H. (1991). 'Premiums without benefits: waste and inefficiency in the commercial health insurance industry', *International Journal of Health Services*, xxi, 2, 265–83.

British Medical Association (BMA) (1993). *The New Health Promotion Package*, London, General Medical Services Committee of the British Medical Association.

British Medical Association and Pharmaceutical Society of Great Britain (twice annually). *British National Formulary*, London, BMA and the Pharmaceutical Press.

Broome, J. (1987). 'Good, fairness and QALYs', in Bell, M. and Medus, S. (eds) *Proceedings of the Royal Institute of Philosophy Conference on Philosophy and Medical Welfare*. Cambridge, Cambridge University Press.

Brownbridge, G., Evans, A. and Wall, T. (1985). 'The effect of computer use in the consultation on the delivery of care', *British Medical Journal*, cclxxxxi, 639–42.

Brownbridge, G., Fitter, M.J. and Sime, M. (1984). 'The doctor's use of a computer in the consulting room', *International Journal of Man-Machine Studies*, xxi, 65–90.

Bullas, S. (1989). *Case Mix Management System Core Specification*. London, NHS Management Board Resource Management Directorate.

Bullas, S., Burford, B. and Lowson, K. (1993). 'System support to community, clinical and general management', in Richards (1993) pp. 45–52.

Burch, J.G. and Grudnitski, G. (1986). *Information Systems, Theory and Practice*. New York, Wiley.

Burdess, C. (1993). 'How to make PRINCE work: success with this new methodology', in Richards (1993) pp. 3–8.

Butcher, R. (1970). 'Social process and power in a medical school', in Zald, M.N. (ed.) *Power in Organisations*. Nashville, Vanderbilt University Press.

Buxton, M., Packwood, T. and Keen, J. (1991). *Final Report of the Brunel University Evaluation of resource management*. Uxbridge, Health Economics Research Group Brunel University.

Calnan, M. (1987). *Health and Illness. The Lay Perspective*. London, Tavistock.

Campling, E.A., Devlin, H.B., Hoile, R.W. and Lunn, J.N. (1993). *The Report of the National Confidential Enquiry into Perioperative Deaths 1991/1992*. London, Royal Colleges of Physicians, Surgeons, Obstetricians and Gynaecologists, Anaesthetists, Pathologists and Radiologists and College of Ophthalmologists.

Carper, W.B. and Litschert, R.J. (1983). 'Strategic power relationships in contemporary profit and nonprofit hospitals', *Academy of Management Journal*, xxvi, 311–20.

Charns, M.P. and Schaefer, M.J. (1983). *Health Care Organisations: A Model for Management*. Englewood Cliffs, Prentice-Hall.

Cherns, A. (1987). 'Principles of socio-technical design revisited', *Human Relations*, xii (1) 153–61.

Chishom, R.F. and Zeigenfuss, J.T. (1986). 'Review of the applications of the socio-technical systems approach to healthcare', *Journal of Applied Behavioral Science*, xxii, 315–27.

Chisnall, P.M. (1991). *The Essence of Marketing Research*. New York, Prentice-Hall.

CIPFA (Chartered Institute of Public Finance and Accountancy) (1987). *Health Service Trends*. London, Healthcare Financial Management Association.

Clayden, D. (1992). 'Information management for health services', Jachranka, Anglo-Polish Health Symposium.

Cochrane, A.L. (1972). *Effectiveness and Efficiency. Random Reflections on Health Services*. London, Nuffield Provincial Hospitals Trust.

Coles, J. (1988). 'Clinical budgeting as a management tool' in Maxwell. R. (ed.) *Reshaping the National Health Service*. Newbury, Policy Journals, pp 126–41.

Cook, K.S., Shortell, S.M., Conrad, D.A. and Morrisey, M.A. (1983). 'A Theory of organisational response to regulation; the case of hospitals', *Academy of Management Review*, viii, 193–205.

Cook, S. (1992). 'Database creation' [review], *Health Education Journal*, li, 2, 150.

Coombes, R.W. (1987). 'Accounting for the control of doctors: management information systems in hospitals', *Accounting, Organisations and Society*, xii, 4, 389–404.

Council of Europe (1981). *Data Protection Convention*. Strasbourg, Council of Europe.

Council of Europe (1991). *Conference on Training Strategies for Health Information Systems, Documents*. Strasbourg, Council of Europe.

Coyne, J.S. (1985a). 'Assessing the financial characteristics of multi-institutional organisations', *Health Services Research*, xix 6, 701–15.

Coyne, J.S. (1985b). 'Measuring hospital performance in multi-institutional organisations using financial ratios', *Health Care Management Review*, x, 4, 35–42.

Cross, M. (1992). 'Indispensable', *Health Services Journal*, 29 October 1992, pp. 33–4.

Cross, M. (1993). 'Hisssssss Bang!', *Health Services Journal*, 17 June 1993, pp. 39–47.

Cruickshank, P.J. (1984). 'Computers in medicine: patients attitudes', *Journal of the Royal College of Practitioners*, xxxiv, 77–80.

Cullen, W. (1769). *Synopsis Nosologiae Methodicae*. Edinburgh: [publisher unknown].

Culyer, A., Maynard, A. and Posnett, J. (1990). *Competition in Health Care: Reforming the NHS*. London, Macmillan.

Cummings, T.G. and Held, E.F. (1985). *Organisation Development and Change*. St Paul, West.

Daniels, A., Turner, M.J. and Gillam, M.T. (1993). 'Costs and benefits of EDI', in Richards (1993) pp. 475–9.

Dawson, S. (1993). 'Pole to pole', *Health Services Journal*, 11 March, 33–4.

De Dombal, F., Leaper, D., Staniland, J. et al (1972). 'Computer-aided diagnosis of acute abdominal pain', *British Medical Journal*, ii, 9–13.

Deming, W.E. (1986). *Out of the Crisis*. Cambridge, Mass., MIT.

Department of Health (1988). *Community Care. Agenda for Action*. London, HMSO.

Department of Health (1989a). *Working for Patients*. London, HMSO.

Department of Health (1989b). *General Practice in the NHS: 1990 Contract*. London, Department of Health.

Department of Health (1989c). *Terms of Service for Doctors in General Practice*. London, Department of Health.

Department of Health (1990a). *NHS and Community Care Act*. London, HMSO.

Department of Health (1990b). *HC(90)15: Medical Audit in the Family Practitioner Services*. London, Department of Health.

Department of Health (1990c). *Working for Patients. Framework for Information Systems: the Next Steps*. London, HMSO.

Department of Health (1990d). *The Care Card – Evaluation of the Exmouth Project*. London, HMSO.

Department of Health (1990e). *Improving Prescribing*. London, Department of Health.

Department of Health (1990f). *Access to Health Records Act*. London, HMSO.

Department of Health (1990g). *Guidelines for Administration of the Access to Health Records Act 1990*. London, HMSO.

Department of Health (1991). *Research for Health: A Research and Development Strategy for the NHS*. London, Department of Health.

Department of Health (1992). *Health of the Nation*. London, HMSO.

Department of Health (1993a). *Making London Better*. London, Department of Health (Tomlinson Report).

Department of Health (1993b). *Managing the New NHS*. London, Department of Health.

Department of Health (periodically). *Statement of Fees and Allowances* London, Department of Health ('Red book').

Department of Health (annually). *Health of the Nation* [data]. London, HMSO.

DHSS (Department of Health and Social Security) (1980). *Inequalities in Health* London, HMSO (Black Report).

DHSS (1982). *Steering Group On Health Services Information. First report to the Secretary of State*. London, HMSO.

DHSS (1983). Letter to Norman Fowler, 6 October 1983: NHS Management Inquiry (first Griffiths Report). London, DHSS.

DHSS (1985). *General Practice Computing, Evaluation of the Micros for GPs Scheme: Final Report*. London, DHSS.

DHSS (1986). *HN(86)34: Health Services Management: Resource Management (Management Budgeting) in Health Authorities*. London, DHSS.

DHSS (1987). *Promoting Better Health: The Government's Programme for Improving Primary Care*. London, HMSO.

Dowling, A., Organisational Issues in Health Informatics Conference, Cincinnati, April 1994 (unpublished).

Downs, E., Clare, P. and Coe, I. (1991). *Structured Systems Analysis and Design Method: Application and Context* 2nd edn. Hemel Hempstead, Prentice-Hall.

Doyal, L. and Gough, I. (1991). *A Theory of Human Need*. Basingstoke, Macmillan.

Eason, K. (1982). 'The process of introducing information technology', *Behaviour and Information Technology*, i, 65–89.

Engels, F. (1975). *The Part Played By Labour in the Transition from Ape to Man*. Beijing, FLPH.

Ernst and Young (1989). *The Landmark MIT Study: Management in the 1990s*, Cleveland/New York, Ernst and Young.

Enthoven, A. (1991). 'The Internal Market Revisited – Information to Support the Internal Market'. IHSM Conference, London, 25 January.

Evans, J. (1993). 'Purchasers' preoccupations revisited', *The Health Summary*, **x**, 2, February, 13–4.

Fairey, M. (1993). 'The missing link: the managerial challenge', in Richards (1993) pp. 15–20.

Farr, W. (1856). *Registrar General of England and Wales: Sixteenth Annual Report 1856*. London, Registrar General.

Ferlie, E. and McKee, L. (1988). 'Planning for alternative futures in the NHS' *Health Services Management Research*, **i** 1, 4–18.

Fisher, P.J. and Kitson, A.J. (1993). 'Economic information tools for healthcare managers', in Richards (1993) pp. 525–33.

Fitchett, M. (1991). 'M25 syndrome', *Health Services Journal*, 5 December, pp. 24–5.

Fitter, M.J. (1987a). 'The development and use of information technology in healthcare', in Blackler, F. and Oborne, D. (eds) *Information Technology and People*. Leicester, BPI.

Fitter, M.J. (1987b). 'The impact of new technology on Nurses and Patients' in Payne, R. and Firth-Cozens, J. (eds) *Stress in Health Service Professionals*, Chichester, Wiley.

Fitter, M.J., Evans, A.R. and Garber, J.R. (1985) 'Computers and Audit', *Journal of the Royal College of General Practitioners*, **xxxv**, 522–4.

Fottler, M.D. (1987). 'Health care organizational performance: present and future research', *Journal of Management*, **xiii**, 2, 367–91.

Foucault, M (1973). *The Birth of the Clinic*. London, Penguin.

Frankel, S. and West, R. (ed.) (1993). *Rationing and Rationality in the National Health Service. The Persistence of Waiting Lists*. Basingstoke, Macmillan.

Freidson, E. (ed.) (1963). *The Hospital in Modern Society*. London, Free Press.

Freidson, E. (1970). *Professional Dominance: The Social Structure of Medical Care*. Chicago, Aldine.

Galbraith, J.K. (1974). *Organisational Design: An Information Processing View*. Reading, Mass., Addison-Wesley.

Galbraith, J.K. (1977). *Organisational Design*. Addison-Wesley. Reading, Mass., Addison-Wesley.

Georgopoulos, B.S. (1986). *Organisational Structure, Problem Solving and Effectiveness*. San Francisco, Jossey-Bass.

Gale, R. (1993). 'The Application of Open Architecture to HISS', in Richards pp. 297–302.

Gane, C. and Sarson, T. (1979). *Structured Systems Analysis*. New York, Prentice-Hall.

Glennerster, H., Matsaganis, M. and Owen, P.A. (1992). *A Foothold for Fundholding*, London, Kings Fund.

Goldberg, C., Griew, A., Tristram, C. and Savill, A.W. (1993). 'How to Buy Healthcare' in Richards (ed.) (1993) pp. 617–22.

Goves, J. R., Davies, T. and Reilly, T. (1991). 'Computerisation of primary care in Wales', *British Medical Journal*, **ccciii**, 93–4.

Greenhalgh, C.A. (1986). 'Management Information Initiatives in the NHS', *Public Finance and Accountancy*, **xvi**, 6–8.

Greenhalgh, C.A. and Todd, G. (1985). 'Financial information project: message for the NHS', *British Medical Journal*, **cclxxxx**, 410–11.

Greenhalgh & Co., (1992). *Using Information in Contracting.* Macclesfield, Greenhalgh.

Greenhalgh, C., Peel, V. and Wright, G. (1992). *Caring for the Community in the 21st Century. Integrated Purchasing of Public Services.* Macclesfield, GCL & HSMU.

Griffiths, R. (1984). *NHS Management Enquiry.* Letter of 6 October 1983, under HN 84(13), London, DHSS.

Guardian, The (1991). (Green, S.) 'Warning: this trade could damage your health care', 31 July 1991, p. 19.

Guardian, The (1992). (Mullin, J.) 'Ambulance chief resigns as delays are blamed for deaths', 29 October 1992, p. 1.

Guardian, The (1993a). (Mihill, C.). 'Hospitals to publish waiting list tables', 7 December 1993, p. 8.

Guardian, The (1993b). Report of minister's answer to Parliament on 6 January 1993; reported 7 January 1993, p. 5.

Gutmann, J. and Annandale, S. (1986). *Consumer Relations Training in the NHS.* Bristol, NHSTA.

Hall, R.H. (1985). 'Professional – Management Relations: Imagery versus Action', *Human Resource Management,* **xii** (3), no.2, 227–36.

Ham, C. (1992). 'Contract Culture', *Health Services Journal,* 7 May, 22–4.

Harris, J. (1985). *The Value of Life.* London, RKP.

Harrison, S. (1988). *Managing the National Health Service: Shifting the Frontier.* London, Croom Helm.

Harrison, S., Hunter, D. and Marnoch. G. (1991). *Just Managing – Power and Culture in the NHS.* London, Macmillan.

Health Economics Research Group (1991). *Final Report of the Brunel University Evaluation of Resource Management.* Uxbridge, HERG.

Health Information Strategy Steering Group (1991). *Health Information Strategy for New Zealand.* Wellington, Department of Health.

Hinnings, C.R. and Greenwood, R. (1988). *The Dynamics of Strategic Change.* Oxford, Blackwell.

Hirschheim, R. (1985a). *Office Automation: A Social and Organisational Perspective.* Chichester, Wiley.

Hirschheim, R. (1985b). 'User Experience with and assessment of participative systems design', *Management Information Systems Quarterly,* **viii,** 295–303.

Holland, W.W. (ed.) (1983). *Evaluation of Health Care.* Oxford, Oxford University Press and European Community.

Ifeachor, E.C. (1993). 'Neural networks and their applications to health care', in Abbott, W. (ed.) A.6.11.

Inglis, B. (1983). *The Diseases of Civilization.* St. Albans, Granada.

Institute of Health Services Management (annually), *Yearbook.* London, ISHM.

Irvine, D.H. (1990). *Managing for Quality in General Practice.* London, Kings Fund.

Jackson, C. (1990). 'All hands to the sails', *Health Visitor,* **lxii,** 11, 376–77.

Jackson, M.A. (1983). *Systems Development.* Englewood Cliffs, Prentice-Hall.

Joint Commission for Accreditation of Healthcare Organizations (USA, annually). *Accreditation Manual for Hospitals.* Chicago, Joint Commission for Accreditation of Healthcare Organizations.

Juran, J. (1993). *Quality Planning and Analysis*, London, McGraw-Hill.

Kennedy, I. (1981). *The Unmasking of Medicine*. London, Allen and Unwin.

Kenny, D.J. (1986). 'Information Technology in the NHS', *Information Technology and Public Policy*, v 1, 6–7.

King, W.R. and Rodriguez, J.I. (1991). 'Participative design of strategic decision support systems: an empirical assessment', *Management Science*, xxvii, 6, 717–26.

Klein, H.K. and Hirschheim, R.A. (1987). 'A comparative framework of data-modelling paradigms and approaches', *Computer Journal*, xxx, 1, 8–15.

Körner, E. (1982). *First Report of the Steering Group on Health Services Information*. London, DHSS (Körner Report).

Kropf, R. (1990). Service Excellence in Health Care through the use of Computers. Michigan: Ann Arbor, Health Administration Press.

Laing, W. (annually). *Review of Private Healthcare*. London, Laing & Buisson.

Lamberts, H. and Wood, M. (eds) (1987). *International Classification of Primary Care*. Oxford, Oxford University Press.

Land, F. and Hirschheim, R. (1986). 'Participative systems design: rationale, tools and techniques', *Journal of Applied Systems Analysis*, x, 91–106.

Larson, M.S. (1977). *The Rise of Professionalism*. Los Angeles, University of California Press.

Leitko, T.A. and Szszerbacki, D. (1987). 'Why do traditional OD strategies fail in professional bureaucracies?' *Organisational Dynamics*, xii, 52–65.

L'Express (1991). 'IBM; le declin d'un empire americain', 13 December, pp. 39–41.

Lingren, O. (1992). 'Clinical risk management in health services: a valuable tool for doctors and managers', *The Clinician in Management*, i, 3, 6–8.

Lipsey, D. (1970). *An Introduction to Positive Economics*. London, Weidenfeld & Nicolson.

Luck, M., Lawrence, B., Pocock, B. and Reilly, K. (1988). *Consumer and Market Research in Health Care*. London, Chapman & Hall.

Lyus, S. (1993). 'Executive toys', *Health Service Journal*, 29 April 1993, pp. 40–3.

McCalman, J. and Paton, R.A. (1992). *Change Management. A Guide to Effective Implementation*. London, Paul Chapman.

McCord, J. (1993). 'Using HISS data for health care record', *The International Hospital Federation*, xxviii, 2, 5–10.

McDaniel, R.R., Thomas, J.B., Ashmos, D.P. and Smith, J.P. (1987). 'The use of decision analysis for organisational design: re-organising a community hospital', *Journal of Applied Behavioral Science*, xxiii, 3, 337–50.

McDougall, J. and Brittain, J.M. (1992). *Uses of Information in the NHS*. Loughborough, British Library.

McFarland, D.E. (1979). *Managerial Innovation in the Metropolitan Hospital New York*. New York, Praeger.

Mackintosh, C. and Bradley, P. (1993). 'A management information system for general practice', in Richards, B. (ed.) (1993) pp. 559–66.

Malin, H. (1992). 'Allocating resources at different service levels'. Jachranka, Anglo-Polish Health Symposium.

Malwhinney, B. (1992). Speeches of 18 June and 10 July.

Manuel, G. (1991). 'Craft and Graft Computers; the art of buying a system' *Health Services Journal*, 29 August 1991. pp. 27–8.

Margulies, N. and Black, S.(1987). 'Perspectives on the implementation of participative approaches', *Human Resource Management*, xxvi, 3, 385–412.

Markwell, D. (1993). 'A standard for the registration and identification of coding schemes for EDI', in Richards, pp. 489–96.

Martini, C.J.M., Allan, G.J.B., Davidson, J. and Beckett, E.M. (1977). 'Health indices sensitive to medical care variation', *International Journal of Health Services*, vii, 293–309.

Maslow, A.H. (1972). *The Farther Reaches of Human Nature*. New York, Viking Press.

Maynard, A. (1991). 'Will competition work?' London, IHSM Conference.

Meadows, W.J. (1993). 'The Community Information System Project', in Richards (1993) pp. 60–5.

Miles, C. (1993). 'Market values', *Health Services Journal*, 12 August, 32–5.

Ministry of Health (1965). *The Standardisation of Hospital Medical Records*. London, HMSO (Tunbridge report).

Ministry of Health, Education and Welfare (Netherlands) (1992). *Bereidheid tot Verandering/Readiness to Change* (Dekker Plan).

Mitroff, I.I. and Mason, R.O. (1983) 'Can we design information systems for managing messes? or, why so many management information systems are uniformed', *Accounting, Organisations and Society*, viii, 2–3, 95–203.

Mohrman, S.A. and Ledford, G.E. (1985). 'The design and use of effective employee participation groups: implications for human resource managers', *Human Relations*, xxiv, 413–28.

Mordelet, P. (1992) 'The New 1991 French Hospital Act: autonomy and competition between the public and private hospital sector, the use of private sector management'. EHMA Conference, Karlstad.

Mulkay, M., Ashmore, M. and Pinch, T. (1987). 'Measuring the quality of life: a sociological invention concerning the application of economics to health care', *Sociology*, xxi, 4, 541–64.

Mullen, P. (1992). 'New queues for old', *Health Matters*, Winter 13, 12–13.

Mumford. E. (1972). *Job Satisfaction*. London, Longman.

Mumford, E. (1983a). *Designing Participatively*. Manchester, Manchester Business School.

Mumford, E. (1983b). *Designing Human Systems*. Manchester, Manchester Business School.

Mumford, E. and Wier, M. (1979). *Computer Systems in Work Design – The ETHICS Method*. London, Associated Business Press.

Mumford, E. (1993), *Designing Human Systems for Health Care – The Ethics Method*. Rotterdam, 4C Corporation.

National Audit Office (1990). *Managing Computer Projects in the NHS*. London, HSMO.

National Casemix Office (1993). *Healthcare Resource Groups Version 2 Consultation Document*. Leeds, NHSME.

National Health Service Centre for Coding and Classification (1993). *General Information Version 3*. Leeds, NHSME.

NHSTD (National Health Service Training Directorate) (1991). *The Compendium of Standards and Guidelines for the Use of Standards*. Bristol, NHSTD.

NHSTD (1994), *Just for the Record. A Guide to Record Keeping for Health Care Professionals*. Bristol, NHSTD.

NHSME (National Health Service Management Executive) (1990). *Costing and Pricing Contracts. Cost Allocation Principles (EL(90)173; 5 October 1990)*. London, NHSME.

NHSME (1991a). *Health Service Indicators. Dictionary 1991*. London, NHSME.

NHSME (1991b). *Clinical Profiles of Care Huddersfield*, NHSME–RMI. London, NHSME.

NHSME (1992a). *FDL(92)53*, 11 June. London, NHSME.

NHSME (1992b). *The Data Manual*. London, NHSME.

NHSME (1992c). *Local Voices*, under EL(92)1, 10 January. London, NHSME.

NHSME (1992d). *EL(92)34*, 28 May. London, NHSME.

NHSME (1992e). *FDL(92)49*, 12 June. London, NHSME.

NHSME (1992f). *FDL(92)47*, 20 July. London, NHSME.

NHSME (1993a). *HSG(93)5*, 18 January. London, NHSME.

NHSME (1993b). *Computerisation in GP practices; 1993 survey*. London, Department of Health and the Central Office of Information. London, NHSME.

NHSME (1993c). *FDL(93)83*, 21 May. London, NHSME.

NHSME (1993d). *EL(93)10*, 20 July. London, NHSME.

NHSME-IMG (National Health Service Management Executive Information Management Group) (1992a). *Information Management and Technology Strategy for the NHS*, London, NHSME.

NHSME IMG (1992b). *Benefits Management. Guidelines on Investment Appraisal and Benefits Realisation for Hospital Information Support Systems*. Birmingham, NHSME.

NHSME-IMG (1993a). *General Medical Practice Computer Systems; Requirements for Accreditation*. London, NHSME.

NHSME-IMG (1993b). *Getting Better With Information*. London, NHSME.

NHSME-RM (National Health Service Management Executive Resource Management) (1991). *Clinical Profiles of Care*. London, NHSME.

NHSTA (National Health Service Training Authority) (1985). *Information Management*. Bristol, NHSTA.

NHSTA (1990). *Using Information to Manage Resources*. Bristol, NHSTA.

Neumann, B., Sheaff, R. and Peel, V. (1992). *Costing Issues Arising from the Resource Management Initiative*. London, Department of Health.

Newman, T. and Jenkins, L. (1991). *DRG Experience in England 1981–1991*. London, CASPE.

Northern Regional Health Authority (1994). Developing the market for Acute Services. Newcastle, NRHA.

Oaker, G. and Brown, R. (1986). 'Intergroup relations in a hospital setting a further test of social identity theory', *Human Resources*, **xxxix**, 8, 767–78.

OPCS (Office of Population Censuses and Surveys) (1987). *Classification of Surgical Operations; 4th revision*. London, OPCS.

OPCS (1988). *The Prevalence of Disability Among Adults*. London, HMSO.

OPCS (1988). *The Prevalence of Disability Among Children*. London, HMSO.

Øvretveit, J. (1991). *Total Quality Management in Health Care*. Oxford, Blackwell.

Packwood, T., Keen, J. and Buxton, M. (1991). *Hospitals in Transition. The Resource Management Experiment*. Buckingham, Open University Press.

Parsons, T. (1951). *The Social System*, Glencoe, Free Press.

Parston, G. (1988). 'General Management', in Maxwell, R. (ed.) *Reshaping the National Health Service*. Oxford, Transaction pp. 17–34.

Passmore, W., Petee, J. and Bastain, R. (1986). 'Sociotechnical systems in healthcare: a field experiment', *Journal of Applied Behavioral Science*, xxii, 3, 329–39.

Peel, V. (1994) 'Management Focussed Health Informatics research and education at the University of Manchester. *Methods of Information in Medicine*. (Forthcoming).

Peel, V., Ellis, L., Loeb, J., Atkinson, C., Booth, M., Cottrey, K., Nickson, J., Rea, C. and Walker, M. (1993). *Evaluation of the Clwyd Resource Management Project*. Manchester, HSMU and CSL.

Pennsylvania Health Care Cost Containment Council (PHCCC) (annually). *Hospital Effectiveness Report*. Harrisburg, PHCCCC.

Perrin, J.R. (1987). 'Resource Management and Clinical Budgeting', *Journal of Management in Medicine*, ii, 2, 99–106.

Petee, W.J. and Bastain, R. (1986). 'Sociotechnical systems in healthcare: a field experiment', *Journal of Applied Behavioral Science*, ii, 329–39.

Petit, M. (1989). 'Le Systeme d'Information en Soins Infirmieres', in Roger-France (1989) pp. 88–99.

Pettigrew, A., McKee, L. and Ferlie, E. (1988). 'Understanding change in the NHS', *Public Administration*, lxvi, 297–317.

Pickin, C. and St Leger, S. (1993). *Assessing Health Need Using the Life Cycle Framework*, Buckingham, Open University Press.

Pollitt, C., Harrison, S., Hunter, D. and Marnoch, G. (1988). 'The reluctant managers: clinicians and budgets the NHS', *Financial Accountability and Management*, iv, 3, 213–33.

Powell, M. (1991). 'Contracts of a clinical kind', *Health Services Journal*, 1 August, 18–19.

Pringle, M. (1985). 'Using a computer in the consultation', in Sheldon, M. and Stoddart, N. (eds) *Trends in General Practice Computing*. London, Royal College of General Practioners.

Pringle, M., Robins, S. and Brown, G. (1984). 'Computers in the surgery: the patients view', *British Medical Journal*, cclxxxviii, 289–91.

ProPAC (Prospective Payment Assessment Commission) (1991; and annually). *Medicare and the American Health Care System. Report to Congress*. Washington, ProPAC.

Provan, K.G. (1987). 'Environmental and organizational predictors of adaptation of cost containment policies in hospitals', *Academy of Management Journal*, xxx, 2, 219–39.

Quinn, J.B. (1980). *Strategies for Change: Logical Incrementalism*. Irwin, Ill, Addison Wesley.

Quinn, J.B. (1992). *Intelligent Enterprise*. New York, Free Press.

Rado, G. (1992). 'Sweden's health care system. The managerial contribution to improved health status', EHMA Conference, Karlstad 1992.

RCS (Royal College of Surgeons of England) (1991). *Guidelines for Surgical Audit by Computer*. London, RCS.

Rae, C. (ed.) (1993). *Managing Clinical Directorates*. Harlow, Longmans.

Raelin, J.A. (1985). 'The basis for the professional's resistance to managerial control', *Human Resource Management*, ii, 147–75.

Redmayne, S., Klein, R. and Day, P. (1993). *Priorities in Hard Times*. Bath, University of Bath Centre for the Analysis of Social Policy.

Registrar General of England and Wales (1856). *Sixteenth Annual Report*. London, Registrar General.

Reuler, J.B. and Balazs, J.R. (1991). 'Portable medical records for the homeless mentally ill', *British Medical Journal*, ccciii, 446.

Richards, B. (ed.) (1988). *Current Perspectives in Healthcare Computing 1988*. Weybridge, British Computer Society.

Richards, B. (ed.) (1993). *Current Perspectives in Healthcare Computing 1993*. Weybridge, British Computer Society.

Richards, B. (1994). *Current Perspectives in Healthcare Computing 1994*, Weybridge, British Computer Society.

Robinson, R. (1991). 'Roll-call after roll-out', *Health Services Journal*, 6 June, 18–19.

Roger-France, F.H., De Moor, G., Hofdijk, J. and Jenkins, L. (eds) (1989). *Diagnostic Related Groups in Europe*. Ghent, UZ Dienst Medische Informatia.

Roger-France, F.H. (1993). 'The road to standards', *Health Informatics Europe*, i, 4, 9–10.

Rooney, M. (1988). 'A proposed quality system specification for the National Health Service', *Quality Assurance*, xiv, 2, 45–53.

Roos, N.R., Schermerhorn, J.R. and Roos L.L. (1974). 'Hospital performance: analyzing power and goals', *Journal of Health and Social Behaviour*, June 1974, xv, 78–92.

Rothman, R.A., Schwartzbaum, A.M. and McGrath, J.H. (1971). 'Physicians and a hospital merger: patterns of resistance to organizational change', *Journal of Health and Social Behaviour*, xii, 46–55.

Royal College of General Practitioners (1980). *Computers in Primary Care: The Report of the Computer Working Party; Occasional Paper No.13*. London, Royal College of General Practitioners.

Royal Commission on the National Health Service (1979). *Report*. London, HMSO.

Sashkin, M. (1984). 'Participative management: an ethical imperative', *Organisational Dynamics*, Spring, ix, 5–22.

Schultz, R.I. and Harrison, S. (1986). 'Physician autonomy in the Federal Republic of Germany, Great Britain and the United States', *International Journal of Health Planning and Management*, 5, 335–55.

Scott, W.R. (1982). 'Managing professional work: three modes of control for health organisations', *Health Services Research*, xvii, 213–40.

Scrivens, E. (1985). '*Policy, power and information technology in the National Health Service*', Bath, University of Bath Social Policy Working Paper.

Scrivens, E. (1987). 'The information needs of district general managers in the English National Health Service', *International Journal of Information Management*, vii, 147–57.

Seabrook, W.H.J. (1993). 'Disaster planning in the NHS', in Richards, pp. 29–34.

Seng, C., Lessof, L. and McKee, M. (1993) 'Who's on the fiddle', *Health Services Journal*, 7 January 1993, 16–17. (see also *The Health Summary*, x, 2, February).

Sheaff, R. (1991). *Marketing for Health Services*. Buckingham, Open University Press.

Sheaff, R. and Peel, V. (eds) (1993). *Best Practice in Health Care Commissioning.* Harlow, Longmans.

Silverman, D. (1970). *The Theory of Organisations.* London, Heinemann.

Smee, C. (1992). *Effect of Tobacco Advertising on Tobacco Consumption: A Discussion Document Reviewing the Evidence.* London, Department of Health Economics and Operational Research Division.

Smith, H.L. (1955). 'Two lines of authority: the hospital's dilemma', *Modern Hospital,* lxxxiv, 59–64.

Starbruck, W.H. and Nystrom, P.C. (1981). 'Designing and understanding organisations', in Starbruck, W.H. and Nystrom, P.C. (eds) *Handbook of Organisational Design.* Oxford, Oxford University Press.

Stewart, F. (1985). *Planning to Meet Basic Needs.* London, Macmillan.

Stoelwinder, J.U. and Clayton, P.S. (1978). 'Hospital organisation development: changing the focus from "better management" to "better patient care"', *Journal of Applied Behavioral Science,* xv, 3, 400–14.

Stokes, A.V. (1993). 'Networking and telecommunications', in Abbott (1993) A6.3.

Szymanski, R.A., Szymanski, D.P., Morris N.A. and Pulschen, D.M. (1988). *Introduction to Computers and Information Systems.* Columbus, Merrill.

Thompson, D. (1987). 'Coalitions and conflict in the NHS: Some implications for general management', *Sociology of Health and Illness,* ix, 2, 127–53.

Tichy, N.M. (1977). *Organisational Design for Primary Care.* New York, Praeger Holt.

Tichy, N.M. (1978). 'Diagnosis for complex health care delivery systems: a model and case study', *Journal of Applied Behavioral Studies,* xiv, 3, 305–20.

Tricker, R. (1983). *Effective Information Management.* Oxford, Beaumont Executive Press.

Twaddle, S. (1993) 'Priority', EHMA conference, Warsaw, 2 July.

US National Committee on Professional and Hospital Activities (US-NCPHA) (1986). *International Classification of Diseases; 9th revision, Clinical Modifications, Annotated edition.* Washington, NCPHA.

Wagner, A. (1993). 'Marketing and market research', in Sheaff and Peel (1993) 3.3.

Wain, R.A. and Holton, S. (1993). 'Experiences with the PHIS model: a systematic approach to purchasing', in Richards (1993) pp. 631–6.

Waldegrave, W. (1991). Announcement to parliament, 21 October 1991.

Wallhouse, R. (1993) 'Successfully integrating information systems into healthcare'. *World Hospitals,* xxviii, 1, 5–6.

Watkins, S. (1987). *Medicine and Labour. The Politics of a Profession.* London, Lawrence & Wishart.

Weed, L.L. (1969). *Medical Records, Medical Education and Patient Care; the Problem Oriented Record as a Basic Tool.* Cleveland, Press of Case Western Research University.

Weick, K.E. (1979). *The Social Psychology of Organising.* New York, Addison-Wesley.

Weiner, J.L., Boyer, E.G. and Farber, N.J. (1986). 'A changing health care decision making environment', *Human Relations,* xxxix, 7, 647–59.

Weisbord, M. (1976). 'Why organisational development hasn't worked (so far) in medical centres', *Health Care Management Review,* viii Spring, 17–28.

Weisbord, M.R., Lawrence, P.R. and Charns, M.P. (1978). 'Three dilemmas of academic medical centres', *Journal of Applied Behavioral Science*, **xiv**, 3, 284–304.

Weisbord, M.R. and Stoelwinder, J.V. (1979). 'Linking physicians, hospital management cost containment and better medical care', *Health Care Management Review*, Spring, **xiii**, 7–13.

Welch, N. (1993). 'Informed decision making', *British Journal of Healthcare Computing*, **x**, 4, 17–18.

Welsh Office NHS Directorate (1990a). *The Welsh Health Planning Forum. Protocol for Investment in Health Gain – Cancers*. Cardiff, Welsh Health Planning Forum; and subsequent protocols.

Welsh Office NHS Directorate (1990b). *Information and Information Technology for the NHS in Wales: Technical Strategy and Implementation Programme*. Cardiff, Welsh Office.

Westcott, P. (1993) 'Contractual Procedures' in Abbott (1993), A.4 2.1, 1–24.

Wilkin, D., Hallam, L. and Doggett, M.A. (1992). *Measures of Need and Outcome for Primary Health Care*. Oxford, Oxford University Press.

Wilson, C.R.M. (1987). *Hospital Wide Quality Assurance*. Ontario, W.B. Saunders.

Winston, C. (1986). *Introducing Körner*. Weybridge, British Journal of Healthcare Computing Publications.

Woodward, J. (1958). *Management and Technology*. London, HMSO.

Woodward, J. (1965). *Industrial Organisation. Theory and Practice*. London, Oxford University Press.

WHO (World Health Organisation) (1977). *International Classification of Procedures in Medicine*. Geneva, WHO.

WHO (1977). *Manual of the International Statistical Classification of Diseases, Injuries and Causes of Death, 9th revision*. Geneva, WHO.

WHO (1984). *Health For All 2000*. Geneva, WHO.

WHO (1986). *Intersectoral Action for Health*. Geneva, WHO.

WHO (1988). *Informatics and Telematics in Health. Present and Potential Uses*. Geneva, WHO.

WHO (1992). *International Statistical Classification of Diseases and Related Health Problems 10th revision*. Geneva, WHO.

Wright, M. (1985a). 'Managing the Introduction of IT in a Not-for-Profit Service Organisation', *International Journal of Operations and Production Management*, **v**, 3, 12–25.

Wright, M. (1985b). *Manage IT! Exploiting Information Systems for Effective Management*. London, Frances Pinter.

Yates, L.J. (1983). 'Technology in Nursing', *Nurses Focus*, **v**, 2, 8.

INDEX

References in italic indicate figures or tables

INFORMATION MANAGEMENT IN HEALTH SERVICES
Justin Keen (ed.)

Health services are set on an inexorable drive for more and better information, and are spending millions of pounds on information technology (IT) in an effort to obtain it. But as the need for information becomes ever more pressing, serious problems have come into focus ranging from the difficulties of collecting accurate routine data to understanding the role of information in management and clinical processes.

The book seeks to clarify the nature of the problems surrounding information and IT, and point the way to practical solutions. It is divided into three sections: policy overview; views from within the health service; and the views of academic researchers.

Contents
Section 1: Overview: information policy and the market – Hospitals in the market – Information policy in the National Health Service – Section 2: The practitioner perspective – Operational systems – Managing development: developing managers' information management – Clinical management – Nursing management – Contracts: managing the external environment – Section 3: The academic perspective – Information for purchasing – The politics of information – A social science perspective on information systems in the NHS – Information and IT strategy – Evaluation: informing the future, not living in the past – IT futures in the NHS – Index.

Contributors
Brian Bloomfield, Andrew Brooks, Jane Clayton, Rod Coombs, Bob Galliers, Wally Gowing, Mark Harrison, John James, Justin Keen, Andy Kennedy, Rebecca Malby, Margaret Marion, Jenny Owen, James Raftery, Ray Robinson, Mike Smith, Andrew Stevens.

224pp   0 335 19116 9 (Paperback)   0 335 19117 7 (Hardback)

CONTROLLING HEALTH PROFESSIONALS
THE FUTURE OF WORK AND ORGANIZATION IN THE NHS

Stephen Harrison and Christopher Pollitt

For twenty years, British governments of both the left and right have tried to improve the management of the NHS. But the distinctive contribution of the Thatcher governments of the 1980s has defined this very much in terms of controlling health professionals: doctors, nurses and others. This volume

- offers an explanation of why this approach was adopted
- examines in detail the various methods of control employed
- assesses the consequences for the future of professional work and organization in the NHS.

The book will be of interest to a wide range of health professionals, including nurses, doctors, health authority members and managers and will also be useful for students of social policy and health studies.

Contents

Professionals and managers – Finance for healthcare: supply, demand and rationing – Challenging the professionals – Incorporating the professionals – Changing the environment – The future of managerial and professional work in the NHS – Notes – References – Index.

192pp   0 335 09643 3 (Paperback)   0 335 09644 1 (Hardback)

PATIENTS, POLICIES AND POLITICS
BEFORE AND AFTER *WORKING FOR PATIENTS*

John Butler

The 1989 White Paper *Working for Patients* was the watershed of the Conservative government's policymaking for the future of the British National Health Service. This book examines the political and historical background to the White Paper, its contents and proposals, and the actions and reactions to which it gave rise. The book is written in an accessible and jargon-free style and is aimed at a wide range of readers from various professional and academic backgrounds who are seeking a synoptic and balanced view of this remarkable episode in the history of the NHS.

Contents
Origins – Context – Content – Purposes – Dissent – Prophecies – Implementation – Reflections – References – Index.

160pp   0 335 15647 9 (Paperback)   0 335 15648 7 (Hardback)